HOW TO WRITE A SUCCESSFUL RESEARCH GRANT APPLICATION

A Guide for Social and Behavioral Scientists

HOW TO WRITE A SUCCESSFUL RESEARCH GRANT APPLICATION

A Guide for Social and Behavioral Scientists

Edited by

WILLO PEQUEGNAT AND ELLEN STOVER

National Institute of Mental Health
Rockville, Maryland

PLENUM PRESS • NEW YORK AND LONDON

Library of Congress Cataloging-in-Publication Data

How to write a successful research grant application : a guide for
  social and behavioral scientists / edited by Willo Pequegnat and
  Ellen Stover.
        p.   cm.
    Includes bibliographical references (p.   ) and index.
    ISBN 0-306-44965-X
    1. Proposal writing for grants.   I. Pequegnat, Willo.
  II. Stover, Ellen.
  HG177.H683   1995
  300'.68'1--dc20   95-23003
                                                         CIP

ISBN 0-306-44965-X

Published 1995 by Plenum Press
Plenum Press is a Division of Plenum Publishing Corporation
233 Spring Street, New York, N. Y. 10013

10 9 8 7 6 5 4

Printed in the United States of America

Contributors

Jeffrey M. Aarons
National Institute of Mental Health
5000 Rockville Pike
Building 10, Room B-2L 312
Bethesda, MD 20892

Peter Adler
Department of Sociology
University of Denver
2040 South Rice
Denver, CO 80208

Hortensia Amaro
School of Public Health
Boston University
85 East Newton Street, M-840
Boston, MA 02118

Robyn Dawes
Department of Social and Decision Sciences
Carnegie Mellon University
5000 Forbes Avenue
Pittsburgh, PA 15213

Robert Dunwoody
Office of Scientific Information
National Institute of Mental Health
5600 Fishers Lane, Room 7-89
Rockville, MD 20857

Eleanor Friedenberg
Division of Extramural Activities
National Institute of Drug Abuse
5600 Fishers Lane, Room # 10-42
Rockville, MD 20857

Richard B. Fritz
Department of Sociology and Anthropology
Saint Xavier University
3700 West 103rd Street
Chicago, IL 60655

Paul Goldstein
Department of Epidemiology
School of Public Health
University of Illinois, Chicago
2121 West Taylor
Chicago, IL 60612

Gregory Herek
Department of Psychology
University of California–Davis
Davis, CA 95616

Jeffrey Kelly
Department of Psychiatry
Medical College of Wisconsin
8701 Watertown Plank Road
Milwaukee, WI 53226

Janice Kiecolt-Glaser
Department of Psychiatry
Ohio State University
473 West 12th Avenue
Columbus, OH 43210

Thomas R. N. Lalley
National Institute of Mental Health
5600 Fishers Lane, Room 10C-06
Rockville, MD 20857

Barry Lebowitz
National Institute of Mental Health
5600 Fishers Lane, Room 7-103
Rockville, MD 20857

Raymond P. Lorion
Department of Psychology
University of Maryland
College Park, MD 20742

William Lyman
Department of Pathology
Albert Einstein College of Medicine
1300 Morris Park Avenue
Bronx, NY 10461

Spero M. Manson
National Center for American Indian and Alaska
     Native Mental Health Research
University of Colorado, Health Sciences Center
4200 East Ninth Avenue
Denver, CO 80262

Ali Manwar
Narcotic and Drug Research Inc.
11 Beach Street
New York, NY 10013

Leonard Mitnick
Office on AIDS, Room 10-75
National Institute of Mental Health
5600 Fishers Lane
Rockville, MD 20857

Frank Mucha
Research Foundation of Mental Hygiene
New York Psychiatric Institute
722 West 168th Street
New York, NY 10032

Bryan Page
Department of Psychiatry
University of Miami
1425 N.W. 10th Avenue
Miami, FL 33136

Delores L. Parron
National Institute of Mental Health
Office of the Director
5600 Fishers Lane, Room 17C-16
Rockville, MD 20857

Willo Pequegnat
Office of AIDS Programs
NIMH, Parklawn, Room 10-75
5600 Fishers Lane
Rockville, MD 20857

Judith Godwin Rabkin
Columbia University
College of Physicians and Surgeons
New York State Psychiatric Institute
722 West 168th Street, Box 35
New York, NY 10032

Juan Ramos
NIMH, Parklawn, Room 18-95
5600 Fishers Lane
Rockville, MD 20857

Robert Remien
New York State Psychiatric Institute
722 West 168th Street, Box 35
New York, NY 10032

Sherry Roberts
Office of AIDS Programs
NIMH, Parklawn, Room 10-75
5600 Fishers Lane
Rockville, MD 20857

Hugh Stamper
Division of Extramural Activities
National Institute of Mental Health
5600 Fishers Lane, Room 9-105
Rockville, MD 20857

Ellen Stover
Office on AIDS
NIMH, Parklawn, Room 10-75
5600 Fishers Lane
Rockville, MD 20857

Anselm Strauss
Department of Social and Behavioral Science
University of California, San Francisco
521 Parnassus, 6th Floor
San Francisco, CA 94143

Jose Szapocznik
University of Miami
Center for Family Studies
1425 N.W. 10th Avenue, 3rd Floor
Miami, FL 33136

H. Gerry Taylor
Rainbow Babies & Children's Hospital
2101 Adelbert Road
Cleveland, OH 44106

Janet B. W. Williams
Columbia University
Box 74
722 West 168th Street
New York, NY 10032

Steven Zalcman
National Institute of Mental Health
Office of the Director
5600 Fishers Lane, Room 11-105
Rockville, MD 20857

Preface

The Department of Health and Human Services has identified Acquired Immunodeficiency Syndrome (AIDS) as the foremost public health problem in the United States. The Centers for Disease Control (CDC) report that, as of December 31, 1994, there were 441,528 documented cases of AIDS in this country, and the number is increasing.

AIDS is an illness characterized by a defect in natural immunity against disease. Many more individuals are known to be infected with Human Immunodeficiency Virus (HIV) but do not have symptoms or the defining characteristics of AIDS. The incubation period for AIDS may range from 1 to 10 or more years in adults and 6 months to several years in children. Infected persons appear to be capable of transmitting infection indefinitely, even if they remain asymptomatic.

In order to increase the number of minority investigators conducting research on HIV infection and AIDS, NIMH conducted a 3½-day technical workshop for minority investigators on July 24–27, 1990, in Fairlakes, Virginia. University-based research programs were asked to nominate investigators who were selected on the basis of a referred 10-page prospectus for a proposed research project. This procedure was used because NIMH wanted to be sure that the prospective investigators were established in a research environment that would provide support for their projects. The objectives of the workshop were to help potential investigators to:

- ✔ Understand the federal research system
- ✔ Become knowledgeable about specific NIMH program initiatives and priorities, especially in AIDS research
- ✔ Become aware of the possible grant mechanisms
- ✔ Know the steps in the review process
- ✔ Understand the steps and process of writing a research grant application

The chapters in this book are based on presentations and discussions held during this workshop and at an NIMH-sponsored meeting entitled "Qualitative Analysis of Textual Data." Some of the information across chapters may be redundant, but we have retained this by design. We feel that this will provide an added emphasis for important points and ensure that you receive the message.

This book is comprehensive. If you are an early career investigator, you may benefit from reading each chapter carefully and reviewing the lists to consider in each section while you are preparing your grant. If you are a more seasoned investigator, you may be more selective in the chapters that you read based on what you feel your strengths and weaknesses as an investigator are.

Willo Pequegnat
Ellen Stover

Office on AIDS
National Institute of Mental Health
Rockville, Maryland

Acknowledgments

We would like to express our appreciation to the many individuals who contributed to the development and implementation of the Research Seminar/Workshop on HIV Infection and AIDS, a technical workshop on which this book is based. During the planning phase, many NIMH program staff members were extremely helpful in developing the curriculum and planning the organization of the workshop. We are grateful to all who generously provided their time and expertise.

Special appreciation is due to Armand Checker; Anita Eichler, M.P.H.; Nancy A. Garrick, Ph.D.; Delores Parron, Ph.D.; Sherman Ragland; Juan Ramos, Ph.D.; and Stanley Schneider, Ph.D., who not only contributed to the selection process of the participants, but also participated in the Research Seminar/Workshop on HIV Infection and AIDS. Robert Johnson, M.D.; Jean Noronha, Ph.D.; Walter Sloboda; and Marvin Stein, M.D., discussed problems that they had encountered with research applications as participants in the NIMH AIDS review committee.

We are grateful to Catherine West and Eugene L. Souder from the Technical Services Branch, Office of Scientific Information, NIMH, who provided the design and graphics for the original book.

Susan Kennell and Sherry Roberts, Office on AIDS, NIMH, and Victoria Grier and Kathy Corrigan, The Circle Inc., provided invaluable coordination of various management functions related to the workshop. Judy Ombura deserves special appreciation for the excellent job that she did in providing technical and typing assistance in the final preparation of the manuscript.

The editing of the manuscripts originally presented at the workshop reflects the cooperation and dedication of the workshop participants, who provided information and revisions in a timely fashion. Also, Joseph Alper and Sam Rosenfeld provided invaluable assistance in preparing the manuscripts. Without the participation of the investigators in the Research Seminar/Workshop, this book would not have been possible.

Finally, while this book is focused on NIMH and AIDS research, the principles and recommendations have applicability across the multitude of programs across neuroscience and behavioral and social science research.

Contents

III   Disseminating Your Findings

Federal Commitment to Support Minority and Women Researchers

Delores L. Parron

The National Institute of Mental Health (NIMH) has played a strategic role in developing the entire spectrum of mental health researchers. Without NIMH, we would not have the understanding of mental disorders, improvements in the mental health system, or knowledge about how behavior affects health generally. NIMH has been at the forefront of AIDS research from the beginning of this epidemic and has contributed to an understanding of the cause and effect of HIV infection and AIDS. In addition, NIMH has been in the vanguard of supporting the development of minority and women researchers. An Associate Director for Special Populations was mandated by the 1980 Mental Health Systems Act, the legislation that implemented the recommendation of the President's Commission on Mental Health. Even though the Act was repealed in 1981, the part that authorized this position was not rescinded. I arrived at NIMH in 1983 as the Associate Director for Special Populations with the responsibility to ensure that all of the Institute's programs are responsive to minority concerns. By 1984, Congress had added women as another special population.

We need the help of all researchers to maintain the federal leadership role in both health and mental health research and specifically in AIDS research. NIH is committed to mobilizing the best intellectual, technical, and moral resources over a wide range of knowledge and perspectives, not only to sustain the tradition that we have established, but also to address the challenges that are still before us. One of those challenges is to address the concerns of special populations—women and minorities.

NIH is keenly aware that, if we expect to implement a national research and service effort to conquer mental illness by the year 2000 and to identify effective preventive interventions for HIV infection, we must use the talents of an array of the best scientists. There is concern about the graying of the American scientific community, and the demographics indicate minority and women scientists will be a larger percentage of the work force by the year 2000. Thus, it behooves us to encourage women and minority researchers to become a part of NIH's research community.

This book is intended to introduce potential researchers to the federal research system, especially minorities and women, and to provide guidance on how to be successful in this process. In short, this handbook is intended to demystify the process of having a successful research application supported by NIH.

The Role of Community Service Groups in Research

Juan Ramos

The constituency of NIMH is a two-tiered system. At one level there are researchers conducting studies of community-based populations, while at another level there are service providers maintaining outreach to these same persons. At NIMH, we are hopeful that there will be more collaboration between these two important professional groups.

In addition to a well-developed research protocol, research requires three resources: financial support, staff, and patients, clients, or subjects. Community-based organizations (CBOs) have the good will and knowledge of the people in the community, while academic centers have the money and the staff. Bringing these two forces together can potentially benefit everyone.

Major national mental health organizations, such as the National Council of Community Mental Health Centers, are placing AIDS on their agenda. There is a need for mental health centers to provide mental health services to persons with AIDS and to their family, friends, and loved ones based on research findings.

The National Association of State Mental Health Program Directors is another community organization that has a major role in the AIDS epidemic. They are concerned because the state mental hospitals have become a place where persons with AIDS are being placed. The state mental health care directors realize that in the future there may be an even greater influx of HIV-infected patients into their facilities, and they want to have trained health care workers and proven programs in place.

The National Mental Health Association, which has affiliates at the local and state level, has identified prevention as an area in which it can provide a leadership role in the AIDS arena.

An organization that is very influential in mental illness is the National Alliance for the Mentally Ill (NAMI). They have state and local AMIs all over the country that are composed mostly of parents. They are concerned about the possible HIV infection risk to their children, who may be in a state mental health facility or a private facility. This is a very real concern, as NIMH researchers have documented an approximately 8% infection rate in private mental health facilities in New York.

There is a sense of urgency in a number of mental health organizations, whether it is at the local, state, or national level. As you read this book and begin to plan your research application, I urge you to view these community-based organizations as a potential resource that can not only assist you in gaining access to research populations but can also help you think through your research process and pose questions that will provide answers that allow these groups to better serve their clientele. This kind of collaboration will improve both the research and the service enterprise.

Grantsmanship and the Review Process

This first section provides an overview of NIMH and the review process. Ellen Stover and Willo Pequegnat describe the relationship between the development of an NIMH research initiative and the budgeting process in response to a public health crisis. The next section by Willo Pequegnat discusses the use of Program Announcements (PA) and Requests for Applications (RFA) as a signal to the field of Institute program initiatives. A personal view of the process of "grantsmanship" is provided by Raymond Lorion, who has views from both inside and outside the system. Hugh Stamper discusses the review process from the time you mail your research application until you receive your summary statement and clarifies some of the review procedures. Eleanor Fridenberg, Thomas Lalley, Barry Lebowitz, and Steven Zalcman present features of the research mechanism that should be matched by the researcher and the project. Potential grantees are advised by Spero Manson to conduct an ethnographic study of the funding organization and to evaluate carefully the critical research issue selected for study in order to develop a career based on a program of research. William Lyman reviews the cues that appear in the summary statement and how to interpret not only the priority score and percentile but also some of the terms chosen to describe your proposal. Finally, Sherry Roberts provides an overview of how the award process is conducted and what steps must be undertaken to ensure that your university receives the grant funds. Each author also shares tips on preparing a research application; while some of this may be redundant, it was included because one message may be more salient to you than another one.

Establishing a Research Program in Response to a Public Health Crisis

Ellen Stover and Willo Pequegnat

The National Institute of Mental Health (NIMH) supports both behavioral and neuroscience research focused on HIV infection and AIDS. These studies have been designed to understand how the virus affects the central nervous system and to identify strategies to change high-risk behaviors that place individuals at risk for HIV infection.

While gay men still account for the majority of persons infected with HIV in this country, in the last several years there has been an increase in the number of women, children, and infants with HIV infection. Heterosexual transmission has also increased, particularly among the partners of injection drug users. In the second decade of the disease there is a disproportionate representation among minorities, particularly African-Americans and Hispanics.

As the epidemic has changed in the United States, the NIMH program initiatives have shifted to meet new challenges. Before discussing the current program initiatives, we would like to review the process by which a new program is established and budget justifications are forwarded to Congress each year in order to obtain resources to support research.

Forces in Public Health Policy

There is a direct interaction among the public's perception of a crisis, the availability of resources, and the development of science. Opportunities are a negotiation between what a field is prepared to contribute and the perceived need of society for certain kinds of information and activity. The continued development of scientific issues in AIDS research requires an adequate and stable level of support for well-trained investigators and an ultimate benefit to persons infected with HIV and to society for that support.

Some converging trends in public health policy highlight the richness of the area of AIDS research for continued research contributions to the entire spectrum of public health problems (Chesney, 1993). For example, findings from AIDS research are contributing to the knowledge of CNS aspects of multiple diseases and to behavior change strategies for other public health problems. As we move to an economy that is dominated by services, the human being figures as a larger part of the equation. Understanding the interaction between individual behavior and public health becomes a more critical factor in establishing health policy. Questions of the individual's responsibility and quality of life are emerging as a larger consideration in public policy decisions (Pequegnat-White, 1976).

There is widespread recognition that many past attempts to implement public health policy have not been successful; increased awareness did not lead to effective prevention campaigns. Often not all the available information was brought to bear in the planning and implementation. The need to include the consumer or the ultimate user of a product or service in the decision-making and evaluation process is being recognized by decision makers as the critical link between knowledge and action (Reed and Collins, 1994).

Another trend is the increasing interest in constructing models to anticipate all permutations of a given set of policies. Otherwise, the solution to one problem may provide the genesis for many more. As part of this planning for the future, alternatives need to be laid out so that the choice points are clearly articulated and the cost/benefit ratio or other qualitative heuristic is computed in advance. As Toffler (1970) remarked in *Future Shock,* finding the non-zero-sum solutions to society's pressing problems requires infinite imagination. The collective imagination of an interdisciplinary team, with each member providing a distinct but interlocking viewpoint, may result in the best possible effort in studying behavioral and neuroscience research issues in AIDS.

Development of the AIDS Research Program

The development of the NIMH AIDS program is a clear example of the interaction between society's perceived need for knowledge and services and an Institute's ability to mobilize support for a group of investigators to study a public health problem.

In 1983 NIMH requested and received $200,000 from supplemental funds that were given to the Alcohol Drug Abuse and Mental Health Administration (ADAMHA)[1] to support the few investigator-initiated grants that related to AIDS. From that modest beginning, the Office on AIDS, NIMH has grown to a current budget for fiscal year 1995 of approximately $90 million. (See Table 1 for the history of the growth in support for the NIMH AIDS research program.)

From an historical perspective, the program has grown in response to a national concern about the public health crisis created by HIV infection. In 1981 the Assistant Secretary for Health requested an immediate PHS response to the increasing epidemic. While in basic research there was a tradition of studying viruses, the ability of NIMH to respond to this request was severely limited because the database in behavioral science on sexual behavior was nonexistent. In fact, there has been a phase-out of social and behavioral research, particularly research focused on sexual behavior, so there was not even a cadre of active researchers concerned with sexual behavior that could immediately be consulted.

---

[1] Editors' note: Congress abolished this agency as of October 1, 1992.

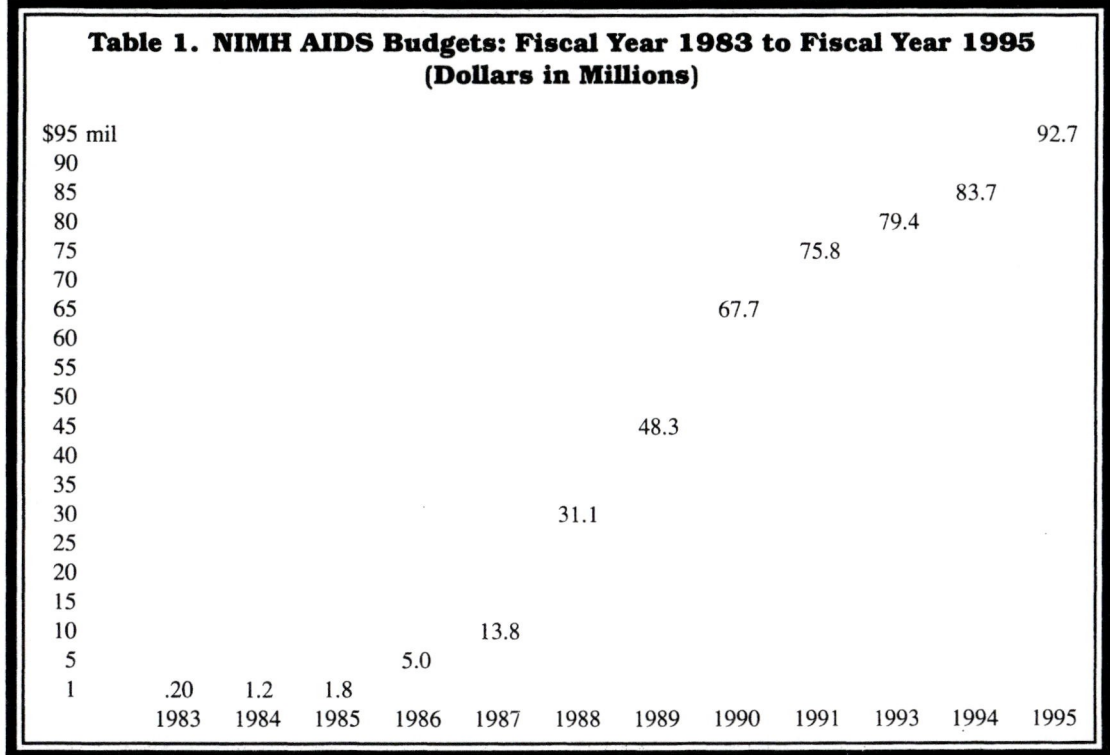

Table 1. NIMH AIDS Budgets: Fiscal Year 1983 to Fiscal Year 1995 (Dollars in Millions)

$95 mil												92.7
90												
85											83.7	
80										79.4		
75									75.8			
70												
65								67.7				
60												
55												
50												
45								48.3				
40												
35												
30								31.1				
25												
20												
15												
10						13.8						
5					5.0							
1	.20	1.2	1.8									
	1983	1984	1985	1986	1987	1988	1989	1990	1991	1993	1994	1995

Role of Consultants

NIMH immediately began to assemble an interdisciplinary group of consultants who were working in allied research areas in behavior and neuroscience in order to build in accountability and credibility for the program. As part of this process of setting goals for the program, a wide range of individuals and organizations were consulted in order to gain a multidisciplinary perspective. Consultations were not limited to academics but were also open to policy specialists, service providers, and persons with AIDS, who were asked to identify critical research issues. These consultants were invited to the Institute, and NIMH program staff made presentations at meetings and conferences. On the basis of this extensive consultation process, interim and long-range goals were established for the program.

Program Staff

In addition to the consultants necessary to establish an effective research program in response to a public health crisis, it is essential that a well-trained staff is recruited to address public health priority areas so that mid-course corrections can be made in response to changing conditions. While the program staff should have a knowledge base, it is equally important that they be able to evaluate information and make a fair decision based on competing needs and opinions.

Peer Review

When a new program is established, it is essential to peer review not only all grants and contracts but also the program concepts on which the first Program Announcements are based. This ensures that the initial calls to the field are viewed as scientifically credible in order to stimulate submission of applications. In addition to ensuring that the program is accountable and credible, the peer review system can also enhance visibility of a new program initiative. Scientists who peer review the program will discuss its goals with colleagues, which is an effective way to increase the number of applications that are received early in the process. In addition, these scientists may also submit grants.

In order to maintain a balance between the need to establish a program of research quickly and to maintain credibility and fairness of the program, Congress mandated expedited peer review for all AIDS grants. Literally, this requires that an application be referred, reviewed, and a decision to fund or not fund made within six months; usually this process takes one year.

Program Announcement (PA) or Request for Applications (RFA)

After program staff members have consulted with the field and established program goals, the Program Announcement (PA) or Request for Applications (RFA) is a signal back to the field about Institute research priorities. There is a specific process that takes approximately one year that must be followed within the PHS system for establishing either a PA or a RFA. It must have Institute approval and must be published in the NIH guide. In addition, other Institutes must be given the opportunity to become a part of any PA or RFA that is directly related to their mission.

A critical decision is deciding whether to issue a PA or an RFA, and there are pros and cons to each. The PA has multiple receipt dates; in the case of AIDS, this is January 2, May 1, and September 1 each year. Once a PA is issued it remains active. The purpose of the PA tends to be broad and to provide research areas as suggestions rather than selection criteria. However, there is no money specifically set aside to fund grants that are submitted under the PA, and these grants are funded from the general extramural research budget.

The RFA, on the other hand, has funds set aside exclusively to fund grants that are submitted in response to it. It is therefore attractive to potential investigators because they feel that this increases their chance of being funded and they may be more likely to respond. However, its purpose may be limited and the investigator may be more constrained in designing his or her study and must meet selection criteria in order to receive funding. Because there is only one receipt date, the staff is gambling that the initial round of applications will be scientifically rigorous, because it will be many months before another solicitation can be released.

Research Mechanism[2]

Another critical area where decisions need to be made early in establishing a new program involves the best mechanisms to meet the program objectives. A well-balanced research portfolio will not only fund a

---

[2] See also "Selecting the Appropriate Research Mechanism" by Friedenberg *et al.,* this volume.

Table 2. National Institute of Mental Health Active AIDS Grants Awards, by Mechanism, September 30, 1993 (Dollars in Thousands)[a]

Research		Number	Total Cost
Research Project Grants		99	32,007
Careet Awards		10	933
Cooperative Agreements		9	5,473
Small Grants		4	277
Conference Grants		1	20
Program Projects		1	1,364
Research Centers		4	15,420
First Awards		5	500
Merit Awards		1	182
		134	56,176
Training	FTTPS		
Individual	7	7	108
Institutional	135	29	3,562
Marc	1	1	24
		37	3,694
Totals		143	59,870

[a] This is an example of the way that the program is distributed by research mechanism and it may vary slightly from year to year.

range of research areas but will also utilize a number of different mechanisms. (See Table 2 for the range of mechanisms that were supported in fiscal year 1993 in AIDS.) In a research area where there is an inadequate database and few well-trained researchers, research centers can be important. These centers can be beacons to others about state-of-the-art research strategies, and they can provide a critical mass of researchers who can benefit from the intense interaction. However, if the initial budget for the program is small, a center can represent a disproportionate percentage of the available support.

Partnership with Referral and Review

During the process of developing a program, the staff in the Division of Extramural Activities (DEA) that has the responsibility for scientific review participates in the development of the final Program Announcement of the submitted research applications. They are instrumental in establishing the schedule for the review of the submitted applications, and they must identify experts who can serve as reviewers. It is also important to establish the referral guidelines so that applications submitted in response to a PA are referred to the appropriate NIMH review committee. DEA is essential in ensuring the scientific integrity of the research and in maintaining the fairness of the process, both of which are critical for continued public acceptance for a research area.

**Table 3. NIMH Fiscal Year 1993
AIDS Budget, by Program Area
(Dollars in Thousands)[a]**

Extramural Research[b]	56,176
Intramural Research	8,328
Research Training	3,694
Research and Development Contracts	6,249
Research Management and Support[c]	3,986
Total	78,433

[a] When NIMH rejoined the NIH in October 1992, the Health Care Worker Program was transferred to SAMSHA, and the NIMH AIDS budget was decreased by approximately $3 million dollars.

[b] Extramural research is the support provided to investigators outside of the Institute at universities and other institutes. Intramural research, on the other hand, supports research conducted by investigators working within the Institute.

[c] This covers the costs of conferences and meetings to review research programs and to identify gaps in current research as well as other program activities.

Grant Monitoring

Most AIDS grants are assigned a Project Officer within the Office on AIDS at the time of submission. This person can provide technical and scientific advice after you receive your summary statement or will monitor your grant application when you receive support. In some cases, if the program person who provided technical assistance in the development of your research application is in one of the three divisions of NIMH, that person may be designated to monitor your grant.[3]

Budgeting Process

At any given time there are multiple budget cycles occurring simultaneously. For example, the federal fiscal year begins on October 1. Thus, during the fourth quarter in 1993 (July, August, and September), the actual expenditures for fiscal year 1993 were being computed, fiscal year 1994 was being approved, the budget for fiscal year 1995 was being marked up by Congress, and budget initiatives for 1996 were being developed by NIH Institutes. (See Table 3 for the proposed 1993 budget.)

---

[3] The three divisions are: Division of Basic Brain and Behavioral Sciences (DBBS), Division of Clinical Research (DCR), and Division of Applied and Services Research (DASR). See also "The Award Process" by Roberts, this volume, on the award process for the branches within the divisions and telephone numbers.

After a program has been established, annual budget justifications are based on the findings or breakthroughs from the previous year. The budget projections are calculated on the actual expenditures for the previous year and the program initiatives for the coming year. In building a program in an area where there is not an established group of investigators or a base of research, initial budgets should include a request for funds that permit pilot testing in new areas. In 1983, when NIMH was asked for a budget proposal for fiscal year 1984, the base was three ROls (individual research grants) and a small grant. It is often difficult to project in advance what areas of science will ultimately be productive. Therefore, it is important to include a range of areas where research can address critical questions.

Program Initiatives

We would like to review the program initiatives of the Office on AIDS as an example of how a program is shaped by forces operating in the public health arena. (Table 4 provides information on the NIMH AIDS budget categories and the actual expenditures in fiscal year 1995.) Each year, meetings are held with NIMH Principal Investigations in order to review the research findings in different areas and to identify promising directions for future research. These are reported to Congress, which ultimately recommends future budgets on the basis of the benefit to the public health from past research support.

The research portfolio is distributed over 15 research mechanisms and is balanced among behavioral and neuroscience research grants (NIMH, 1994). About half the effort is devoted to behavioral research, while the other half is directed to efforts in neuroscience. Approximately 11%, or $7.3 million, is devoted to intramural AIDS research.

Many of these initiatives involve staff from one or more divisions and offices. Program staff from the Office on AIDS work closely, for example, with the Office of Special Populations, and the Deputy Director for Prevention on a variety of initiatives focused on increasing the number of minority PIs and on prevention research in minority populations. NIMH AIDS program initiatives also involve extensive

---

Table 4. NIMH Fiscal Year 1995 AIDS Expenditure, by Budget Categories (Dollars in Thousands)[a]

Natural History and Epidemiology	11,633
Etiology and Pathogenesis	25,593
Therapeutics	5,505
Behavioral Research	42,025
Training and Infrastructure	3,961
Information Dissemination	718
Total	89,435

[a] The 1993 budget has been converted into the new budget categories established by the NIH Office on AIDS Research which were officially adopted by NIMH in fiscal year 1995. The new categories are: Epidemiology and Natural History, Pathogenesis, Therapeutics, Vaccines, and Behavioral.

inter-Institute collaborations within the National Institutes of Health (NIH) as well as intra-agency collaborations with the Centers for Disease Control (CDC), Health Resources and Services Administration (HRSA), and Substance Abuse Mental Health Services Administration (SAMSHA). NIMH has developed a research strategy entitled "AIDS Research: An NIMH Blueprint for the Second Decade." This document discusses past accomplishments and lays out research opportunities and questions for the future. The following section discusses those areas.

Neuroscience Issues in HIV Research

The human immunodeficiency virus (HIV-1) infects cells in both the immune system, particularly CD4+ T-lymphocytes, and the brain. Individuals with AIDS often exhibit neurological and behavioral deficits in addition to profound immunological deficiencies. The effects of HIV-1 on the brain and the immune system, however, are not independent. For example, macrophages are present in the HIV-1–infected brain in large numbers. In addition, the brain and immune system are linked by a variety of neural and hormonal signals, some of which may be altered by HIV-1 infection. Although progress has been made in studying the neuroscience of HIV-1 infection and AIDS, answering important research questions in this area remains an important priority area.

Both direct and indirect mechanisms have been postulated to be associated with mental dysfunction in HIV-infected individuals. Determining whether or not replication of HIV directly causes impairment of mental functions is an important area of research. Well-controlled studies of such functions and measurement of viral load in the CNS of HIV-infected individuals as a function of anti-viral therapy (e.g., those treated with AZT) need to be conducted.

A discrepancy exists between the presence of detectable HIV and neuropathologic lesions in the postmortem brain in individuals with AIDS. This discrepancy may be due to either insensitivity of methods for virus detection or lack of a causal relationship between HIV and the lesions in brain. Another important area of investigation uses systematic morphometric measurements of HIV by sensitive novel methods such as *in situ* polymerase chain reactions to correlate with pathologic lesions in brains of HIV-infected individuals not treated with anti-viral drugs and not having opportunistic pathogens in the CNS.

There is concern about the extent to which the brain is a reservoir of HIV-1 and the process by which latent virus affects the brain. A priority area is studying whether the CD4 molecule serves as a receptor for HIV-1 in the brain as it does on T-lymphocytes or whether there are other molecules in the brain that might act as receptors for the virus. The blood–brain barrier is also being studied as a possible target for HIV-1. The role that neurotoxins play in neurological damage produced by HIV-1 infection is being reviewed. Further, there is a question about whether the life cycle of HIV-1 differs in brain and systemic infections.

The development of a variety of animal models is essential in studying the behavioral and neurological changes that occur both during and after infection and in developing potential therapies for treating and preventing HIV infection. The models being developed under the auspices of NIMH, both intramural and extramural, are aimed at elucidating the mechanisms by which viruses similar to HIV-1 infect the brain and at assessing behavioral changes that occur in animals infected with HIV-1 itself or related viruses. There is interest in studying the differences and similarities between the CNS dystrophy in infantile and AIDS dementia complex in juvenile and adult animal models; there is uncertainty about whether they represent different disease processes or manifestations of the same underlying pathophysiological mechanisms.

NIMH-supported investigators are initiating studies to address these priority areas. The results of future studies may provide further clarification of the mechanisms that contribute to neurological and behavioral changes that accompany infection with HIV-1 (Pequegnat, Garrick, & Stover, 1992).

Neurobehavioral Issues in HIV Research

Because HIV infection of the CNS occurs frequently and early in the course of the disease, neurobehavioral assessment is important in identifying early symptoms of HIV infection. These assessments can provide valuable information on neurocognitive dysfunction related to HIV that can provide the basis for prevention and treatment. Neuropsychological assessment can be used either as a predictor or mediator of behavior or as a clinical endpoint in the evaluation of the efficacy of new drugs in preventing or reversing AIDS-related cognitive dysfunction.

NIMH convened a group of experts in neuropsychological assessment to make recommendations on an adult battery that would be sensitive to early cognitive changes associated with HIV infection. This group recommended an NIMH battery that evaluates domains. This group also recommended inclusion, to the extent possible, of evaluation of psychiatric status and emotional functioning (Butters *et al.*, 1990).

Emerging findings point to the potential utility of psychiatric medications for HIV-related mental disorders. However, serious gaps in knowledge exist regarding the association between HIV-1 infection and the development of psychopathology (hypomania associated with AZT) and the interactions of psychiatric drugs and HIV therapeutics (AZT and treatments for pneumonia and opportunistic infections). Another major unknown is the effect of low versus high doses of AZT on cognitive decline.[4] NIMH will continue to give priority to research that identifies neuropsychological deficits and relates them to everyday functioning and disease progression. A clinical trial is required to develop an assessment strategy to diagnose these conditions and test the efficacy of unique therapeutics for treating some of these conditions.

NIMH has played a key role in the development of a number of initiatives related to the detection and assessment of neurodevelopment in infants and children. In infants and children the most frequent manifestations of this disease include cognitive deficits, developmental abnormalities, acquired microcephaly, and bilateral corticospinal tract signs that are progressive in a majority of children (Belman, 1991). In pediatric studies, neurodevelopmental changes are increasingly being used to test the efficacy of pharmacological and psychosocial interventions. NIMH has developed a Neuropsychological and Neurological Assessment Battery for Infants and Children to be used to evaluate neurodevelopmental changes in longitudinal pediatric studies. This assessment battery is being field tested in research study ACTG 188 as part of the AIDS Clinical Trials Group (ACTG) in collaboration with NICHD (National Institute of Child Health and Human Development) and NIAID (National Institute of Allergy and Infectious Disease).[5] At the conclusion of this study, investigators will have potent tools to test the efficacy of both educational and psychopharmacologic interventions on HIV disease progression in children.

NIMH will provide support for the expanded use of both the adult and pediatric assessment batteries developed under its auspices.

---

[4] A clinical trial is required to develop an assessment strategy to diagnose these conditions and test the efficacy of unique therapeutics for treating some of these conditions.

[5] See also the discussion of pediatric AIDS on pages 21–22 in this chapter.

Primary Prevention Issues in HIV Research

Even though there have been recent medical advances in therapeutic approaches to HIV infection, the identification of effective and efficient strategies to prevent the spread of HIV infection remains a top public health priority. There continues to be a critical need for systematic information that can be used to improve federally funded HIV prevention programs and develop new prevention initiatives.

The urgency of the AIDS crisis demands that priority be given to research with implications for preventive interventions that reduce the incidence of HIV infection. Even if a vaccine were to be identified in the next few years, prevention efforts would continue to be the primary way to prevent the further spread of HIV-1 infection. A secondary prevention goal is to prevent excess disability in those individuals already infected, such as minimizing depression, anxiety, or cognitive disorders and to promote effective coping with the disease itself and bereavement.

The NIMH plays a unique role in the PHS through supporting research and training to prevent the further spread of HIV. (See Table 5 for the philosophy of the NIMH prevention initiative.) Currently a priority area is studying preventive interventions at three levels: (1) individual/small group, (2) institutional, and (3) community. NIMH is also interested in funding studies that examine the role of the family in preventing and adapting to HIV infection. Most findings to date are from studies of individuals and small groups of individuals at high risk for acquiring HIV. Although some notable studies have demonstrated the effectiveness of the community interventions, this is an approach that needs further research (Kelly *et al.*, 1992).

One example from a study in Miami funded by NIMH is illustrative. Ethnographic researchers have shown that the critical variable in changing drug-using practices in shooting galleries is the behavior of the owner of the gallery. If he/she establishes certain norms, such as requiring needles to be cleaned, this will have an impact on the behavior of those using this shooting gallery and will lower the HIV risk for the patrons of the gallery.

Preventing or changing high-risk behaviors and maintaining low-risk behaviors has been a major area of support. Current work in the prevention of HIV infection has identified some major strategies that can improve the effectiveness of interventions.[6] Prevention programs should be integrated into ongoing systems of care (e.g., STD clinics, family medicine clinics, etc.) and into institutions where hard-to-reach individuals at high risk can be contacted without requiring them to come to prevention programs.

While effective programs will continue to be targeted at the schools, another major initiative is the development of intervention strategies that can be used in workplaces and other community-based institutions, such as PTAs, churches, service clubs, and others.

Another major initiative is with prison populations, where seroprevalance rates have been documented at a level above the national average. Many prisoners have a history of high-risk behavior associated with HIV infection transmission. Preventive interventions designed for this incarcerated population with unique problems will be a critical area of investigation.

Cross-cultural variables deserve special consideration because of the rapidly increasing rates of HIV-1 infection in ethnic minority populations. In such research, operational definitions of cultural factors need to move beyond merely identifying people according to researcher-defined social categories (e.g., race and gender) and should include culturally relevant constructs and assessments (Pequegnat *et al.*, under review).

Prevention research has been fostered by NIMH through the establishment of AIDS research

---

[6] See "Designing an Intervention Study" by Szapocznik and Pequegnat, this volume.

Table 5. AIDS Prevention: Research and Practice

Promoting collaboration to improve research, services, and AIDS education
Facilitating the transfer of research findings to clinical and community settings
Facilitating the transfer of clinical and community experience to research studies

---

centers; currently the prevention ones are in New York, San Francisco, and Milwaukee. Behavioral scientists have designed a range of interventions based on collecting knowledge, attitude, and behavior data during Phase I, Phase II, and Phase III studies. In addition, this center has made critical links to researchers in the AIDS Clinical Trials Group (ACTG) system and will be exploring behavioral factors relevant to adherence in clinical trial protocols.

NIMH-supported preventive intervention studies show remarkable convergence among the major components of successful behavior change strategies. However, most of these results were obtained using only a single site with few subjects and therefore have poor external validity. Research that tests interventions across multiple populations in diverse geographic settings is critically needed in order the address the changing patterns of the spread of HIV infection in the United States.

In fiscal year 1990, NIMH initiated a cooperative agreement to test systematically prevention approaches across multiple populations and sites. This study was designed and is being conducted at seven sites. The study populations include both males and females as well as different ethnic groups. After the Phase III efficacy data are available, CDC is interested in conducting a Phase IV effectiveness trial with this intervention, Project Light.

Many HIV prevention strategies are based on the cognitive behavior model. While behavioral theory provides an important basis for designing HIV prevention programs, it is important to remember that, in San Francisco, the public health strategy for HIV risk reductions includes additional interventions, such as community organizations, social marketing, and efforts to promote changes in group norms concerning risk-taking behaviors. In the second decade of AIDS research, there are different questions in stemming the spread of HIV infection that should be addressed. Other theories and models of prevention and behavior change that may be effective should be explored. (See Table 6 for future prevention research priorities.)

Secondary Prevention

As more people are diagnosed with AIDS, the importance of preventing symptoms and disease progression becomes greater. There is an extensive literature on the relationship between stress/coping and disease progression in cardiovascular and cancer research. This body of evidence indicates that greater variance in disease progression may be attributed to the patients' experience of stress and coping than to the disease itself (Spiegel *et al.,* 1989). The patient who handles the illness better may have used adaptive coping strategies, thereby minimizing the stressfulness of the illness and maintaining better health status. On the other hand, patients whose initial appraisal of the situation leads to maladaptive coping may increase the experience of anxiety and impede the benefit of the prophylaxis.

Although some experiences can jeopardize quality of life by threatening a person's emotional,

---

Table 6. Future Prevention Research Priorities

Preventing relapse. In many populations (e.g., gay men), there has been unprecedented behavior change. However, the maintenance of that change requires the identification of the determinants of the maintenance of behavior change so that boosters can be built into the intervention.

Institutional approaches. Some activities focus on the schools as a vehicle for preventive intervention programs. In addition, appropriate programs need to be developed for churches, prisons, and other institutions where there is a unique need for prevention efforts.

Family-oriented research. Most primary prevention research focuses on the individual. An initiative is required to stimulate research that utilizes the potential of the family as the mediator of the primary prevention messages and in implementing secondary and tertiary prevention efforts.

Minority investigators. The second decade of AIDS will have a profound effect on ethnic minority communities. It is therefore important that an additional effort be made to develop qualified minority investigators who can serve as PIs on prevention projects in these communities.

Hard-to-reach populations. There is still a need to develop approaches for closeted and other hard-to-reach populations (e.g., undeclared gay and bisexual men, drug users, homeless, mentally ill, sociopaths, etc.).

Women. The special behavioral and psychosocial issues for women that are distinct from those of men need to be identified as the basis for more effective public health prevention programs.

Infants and children. Infants and children who have been exposed to HIV infection early in their development need to have effective secondary and tertiary prevention programs developed. These include both educational and psychosocial interventions.

Rural. In many regions of the country the statistics for HIV infection in rural areas is similar to urban areas, especially in the southeast. However, little attention has focused on the unique approaches that will be required to mount effective programs in rural areas.

Expanding theories, models, and methods. In addition to social learning theory, additional theories need to be developed as the basis for preventive intervention approaches. Data analytic strategies that can handle repeated measures so that spurious results are not reported should be explored.

---

physical, cognitive, or economic functioning, research demonstrates that resilience and effective behavioral and cognitive strategies can ameliorate stressful effects (Chesney, 1993; Folkman, 1991). Coping is a complex process that involves not only problems associated with minimizing the experiences of stress but also maximizing and maintaining valued aspects of quality of life while attempting to adapt to or resolve a situation.

Persons with HIV-1 infection may handle multiple problems, some of which are discrimination, limited financial resources, loss of family members, immediate child care problems during illness and ultimate placement after death, transportation, housing, lack of drug treatment programs for women, pregnancy, educational problems of children, crime in the streets, lack of employment opportunities, social stigma and isolation, crime, and violence, to name only the obvious stressful life events. In addition, persons with HIV infection must handle the medical impact of HIV-1 disease, the lack of coordinated medical care and medication, recurrent hospitalizations, and separation from their social support system.

Counseling Strategies

HIV antibody testing and counseling are considered to be an initial component of an HIV prevention strategy. Previous NIMH-initiatives have focused on broad issues in an effective counseling strategy. The counseling issues that need to be addressed are in delineating the issues and techniques to be used in (1) making the initial decision to be tested, (2) learning results, (3) reducing high-risk behavior, (4) adopting health-promoting activities, and (5) learning coping strategies to handle the effects of being seropositive or at high risk to become seropositive. An important area where more work is required is in the development of guidelines to be used in developing a counseling program.

Family-Oriented Research[7]

In recent years researchers, health professionals, and family practitioners have increasingly recognized the importance of the family in issues of prevention, health, illness, and treatment. HIV infection and AIDS are diseases that affect the entire family, and, unlike other diseases, multiple members of the family may be infected.

A coordinated research effort is needed to identify the services that families need in order to mobilize prevention efforts and to cope effectively with HIV infection and AIDS (see Table 7). In order to plan effective primary and secondary prevention programs for families, it is necessary to address some of the following issues: (1) strategies families use to promote or encourage family members to decrease high-risk behaviors; (2) the impact of socioculturally related factors and family system functioning on issues relevant to the perception of AIDS risk and risk reduction among poor, urban, and ethnic families; (3) the methods discordant couples use to negotiate safer sexual practices;[8] (4) strategies families successfully use to cope; and (5) the significance of support from family and friends in decreasing disease progression and increasing quality of life.

In 1992 NIMH took the lead with NIDA and NIAAA in issuing an RFA to examine family processes, and, in 1995, NIMH took the initiative on an RFA with NIDA, NIAAA, and NIA to develop family-oriented interventions. NIMH convenes an annual conference on the role of the family in preventing and adapting to HIV/AIDS the third week in July.

Seriously Mentally Ill and Homeless

Another priority area is the development of preventive interventions that will be successful with patients who may have compromised mental abilities and who may be severely depressed (Stover and Pequegnat, 1994).

Special populations, such as the seriously mentally ill and homeless, may be at high risk for HIV infection. Results from an NIMH-supported blinded seroprevalence study at a private psychiatric hospital in New York City indicated that 7.1% of 350 consecutively admitted patients were HIV positive (Sacks *et al.*, 1994). Moreover, 64% of the patients with HIV infection were also documented to be engaging in HIV risk-taking behavior. In a study of seriously mentally ill men in a New York shelter, the seroprevalent rate was 19% (Susser 1994).

---

[7] Family is construed to be "diverse networks of mutual commitment."

[8] "Discordant" refers to a couple where one partner is seropositive and the other partner is seronegative.

Table 7. The Role of the Family in Preventing and Adapting to HIV infection

- HIV is a family disease because, unlike other chronic diseases, multiple members may be infected.

- Definitions of family need to be expanded to include the infinite variety of "diverse networks of mutual commitment."

- Issues of ethnicity, culture, gender, sexual orientation, and SES (social and economic status) need to be considered in designing preventive interventions with families.

- It is important to understand the power system in the family and to target the most influential person. Often the person for whom the intervention is planned (the woman who comes to the clinic) is not the person with the power to make real changes in the family or with its individual members.

- In designing preventive interventions, it is important to study families who are handling HIV infection with resilience as well as dysfunctional families.

- Families may mediate the interventions of institutions (e.g., school, work place, social services, churches, etc.), but little attention has been given to the family in designing interventions to be conducted within these institutions.

- The goal of interventions should be "family preservation."

- Any preventive intervention should coordinate the multiple systems that are intervening with the family.

Individuals with HIV infection identified as being highly depressed were more likely to use illicit drugs and engage in high-risk sexual practices, which raises clinical concerns for the infected individual and public health concerns regarding further spread of HIV infection.

Ethnic Minorities

NIMH has made a major commitment to increasing the number of ethnic minority researchers being supported to conduct AIDS research. A technical assistance workshop, which is the basis of this book, was held for ethnic minority investigators in 1990. NIMH also supports a number of ethnic minority investigators under supplements to ongoing grants.[9] A workgroup of NIMH researchers is currently examining issues of cultural sensitivity of existing measures in pediatric populations. This is particularly important in assessing changes in children who are not English-speaking.

Women and AIDS Initiatives

Women still represent a minority of cases of AIDS in the United States, but the number of women infected with HIV-1 is growing at an alarming rate; in fact, the rate of growth is approximately

---

[9] See "Program Announcements and Requests for Applications: Signals to the Field" by Pequegnat, this volume, for a description of this program.

three times that of men. Women may be at higher risk of becoming HIV-1 infected through hetero-sexual intercourse because of the possible greater risk to the receptive partner. The majority of women are of reproductive age and represent a diverse multicultural, multiracial group. At least half of the women may have been injection drug users (IDUs), and about 20 percent are the sexual partners of IDUs.

Although women are an understudied group in AIDS research, there is some preliminary evidence suggesting that women have a different clinical course than men. If this is true, there may be multiple biological, psychological, and social reasons that influence virus exposure and disease progression: (1) difference in hormones and genetics that affect disease pathogenesis, (2) failure to diagnose HIV-1 early in the disease process, (3) inappropriate treatment, (4) inability to access health care systems, or (5) stressors resulting from multiple gender-defined roles.

In designing a natural history study of HIV disease progression in women, it is critical to select the predictive and outcome variables that are gender-specific. Health can be influenced by a wide variety of factors, but certain issues may be unique to women, and psychosocial factors may affect women and men differentially. There are gender differences in role expectations, and often an imbalance exists in the amount of social support women receive in comparison to the amount that they give. Women may therefore experience stress from multiple roles in which they have a lot of responsibility but very little control. The inability to cope with stressful situations may impact negatively on their health and disease progression.

A major initiative of the Office on AIDS is the support of studies to address these issues. The Clinical Trial, NIMH Multisite HIV Prevention Trial, will have sufficient women to examine some of these issues.

Pediatric AIDS

A major obstacle in conducting longitudinal studies with infants and children is the fact that no stan-dardized test spans the ages from birth to 9 years of age. The assessment battery developed by NIMH is construct-driven, so that some statements about neurodevelopment in specific abilities can be made for children, although the instrument on which it is measured may change. In addition, scaling between instruments is being established so that the metric will be comparable and a unit of change on one instrument will be equivalent to a unit of change on another instrument (for example, the BSID-II to the Stanford-Binet IV). A major priority is the continued improvement of assessment methodology for infants and children.

NIMH is also using the NIMH battery in collaborating with the NICHD and NIAID on a meth-odological study of neurobehavioral assessment of infants and children with HIV-1 infection. Because HIV-1 infection of the nervous system occurs frequently and early in the course of the disease with infants and children, this is an unprecedented opportunity to remedy the paucity of assessment methods for preschool children. The proposed developmental approach will permit better understanding of the pathogenesis of the neurologically based behavioral, cognitive, and motor abnormalities observed in these infants and children with HIV-1 infection and AIDS and will allow better assessment of change whether due to growth or to treatment. These neurobehavioral assessments can contribute to research and health care practice with HIV-1-infected children and their families in the following ways: (1) early identification of neurologically based signs of HIV-1 infection, (2) appropriate pharmacologic interven-tions can then be initiated in a more timely fashion, (3) the efficacy of drug therapy can be established by evaluating changes in behavior, and (4) behavioral interventions and educational programs that may benefit HIV-1 infected children can be developed. An additional benefit of this assessment approach is the fact that it is often seen as a positive and motivating aspect of research participation by families.

Health and Mental Health Services Research

NIMH supports research on mental health service needs and the provision of mental health services to persons with HIV infection and mental illness who are in either health or mental health treatment settings. Studies of patterns of clinical care provided in different sectors of the health and mental health systems, including studies of detection, diagnosis, treatment, and referral, are important in providing both primary and secondary HIV prevention services. The role of the family in the prevention of and adaptation to HIV infection is also being stressed. Studies and evaluation of innovative models of mental health service delivery for persons with HIV infection and mental illness are underway as well. The development of methods to facilitate research on persons with HIV who have a history of mental illness or who are seriously mentally ill is important in stemming the spread of HIV in this population. Studies of mental illness severity associated with HIV, measures of mental health services or systems characteristics, measures of direct or indirect services costs, measures of family and caretaker burden, measures of mental health services outcomes, quality-of-care measures, and methodologies for using longitudinal study designs are of special concern to NIMH researchers.

Research Training

In a newly emerging area of research, in addition to soliciting research applications directed to program goals it is important to build a cadre of well-trained researchers. In AIDS this is critical because the problem itself spans several areas of expertise, and so even experienced researchers may need to learn new techniques and approaches. Developing both institutional and individual research training opportunities is therefore an important part of the strategy to respond to a public health crisis.

The first generation of investigators entering a new area of research often consists of broad-gauged persons who have a facility for synthesizing concepts. Although they were well-trained in a particular discipline, they see the implications of their theoretical and methodological expertise for the emerging problems. The second generation is trained in the new area by persons whose primary allegiance is to the parent discipline. This second generation, however, is not as constrained and borrows freely from other disciplines. It is this approach that infuses the area with a "hybrid vigor" that the second generation passes along to the next generation. The third generation may be theoretical mavericks whose position is startling to some members of the first generation, who only sought to apply some of the technology of their discipline to a new area of research (Pequegnat-White, 1976).

Currently, the Office on AIDS is providing support to train second and third generation researchers. Approximately sixteen programs are solely supported by AIDS dollars, while twenty programs receive additional AIDS dollars to support an AIDS component as part of an ongoing training program; both predoctoral and postdoctoral fellows are provided with research training in AIDS.

Every other year a meeting of the behavioral and neuroscience training program directors and several trainees from each site is held to share research directions. In addition to hearing presentations from postdoctoral fellows, the research directors discuss issues of recruitment and retention of fellows and curriculum development. Research training continues to be an important area of support because

AIDS research often requires combining multidisciplinary expertise (e.g., immunology and psychosocial studies).

Conclusion

While basic neuroscience and psychosocial research provided a strong basis for the early studies in AIDS research, AIDS research is now informing other areas of research with its findings and methodological advances (Chesney, 1993). The work that has been supported by NIMH on primary and secondary AIDS prevention research initiatives has provided critical information to other agencies, to individuals at risk or infected, and to policy makers in their fight to prevent the further spread of HIV. The NIMH program initiatives will continue to highlight the major role that NIMH plays in identifying central nervous system effects of HIV infection, clinical issues in HIV-related mental disorders, mental health services research areas related to HIV infection and the severely mentally ill, and effective prevention strategies to change high-risk behaviors.

References

Belman, A. L. 1991. AIDS and pediatric neurology. *Pediatric Neurology 8:* 571–603.

Butters, N., Grant, I., Haxby, J., Judd, L. L., Martin, A., McClelland, J., Pequegnat, W., Schacter, D., & Stover, E. 1990. Assessment of AIDS-related cognitive changes: Recommendations of the NIMH Workshop on Neuropsychological Assessment Approaches. *Journal of Clinical and Experimental Neuropsychological Assessment Approaches 12:* 963–978.

Chesney, M. A. 1993. Health psychology in the 21st century: Acquired Immunodeficiency Syndrome as a harbinger of things to come. *Health Psychology 12:* 259–268.

Folkman, S., Chesney, M., McKusick, L., Ironson, G., Johnson, D. S., and Coates, T. J. 1991. Translating copying theory into an intervention. In: J. Eckenrode, ed., *The Social Context of Stress.* New York, Plenum Press, pp. 239–260.

Kelly, J. A., Muphy, D. A., Roffman, R. A., Solomon, L. J., Winett, R. A., Stevenson, L. Y., Koob, J. J., Ayotte, D. R., Fyn, B. S., Desiderato, L. L., Hauth, A. C., Lemke, A. L., Lombard, D., Morgan, M. G., Norman, A. D., Sikkema, K. J., Steiner, S., & Yaffe, D. M. 1992. Acquired Immunodeficiency Syndrome/Human Immunodeficiency Virus risk behavior among gay men in small cities: Findings of a 16-city national sample. *Archives of Internal Medicine 152:* 2293–2297.

NIMH. 1994. Abstracts of NIMH Grantees. Office of AIDS Program, National Institute of Mental Health, Rockville, Maryland.

Pequegnat-White, W. 1976. Alternative job settings in environment and behavior. In: P. J. Woods, ed., *Career Opportunities for Psychologists: Expanding and Emerging Areas* (pp. 65–82). Washington, DC: American Psychological Association.

Pequegnat, W., Nuttal, E. V., Laosa, L., Garcia Coll, C., Gaiter, J., Rodrigues, E., & Alexandre, A. Multicultural assessment issues in research on neurodevelopment of infants and children with HIV-1 infection and AIDS, under review.

Pequegnat, W., Garrick, N. A., & Stover, E. 1992. Neuroscience findings in AIDS: A review of research sponsored by the National Institute of Mental Health. *Journal of Neuro-Psychopharmacology and Biological Psychiatry 16,* 145–190.

Reed, G., & Collins, B. 1994. Mental health research and service delivery: A three-communities model. *Psychosocial Rehabilitation Journal 17(4):* 69–96.

Sacks, M., Dermatis, H., Burton, W., Hull, J., & Perry, S. 1994. Acute psychiatric illness: Effects on HIV-risk behavior. *Psychosocial Rehabilitation Journal 17(4):* 5–18.

Spiegel, D., Bloom, J. R., Kraemer, H. C., & Gottheil, E. 1989. Effect of psychosocial treatment on survival of patients with metastatic breast cancer. *The Lancet 14,* 888–901.

Stover, E., & Pequegnat, W., eds. 1994. *Psychosocial Rehabilitation Journal 17(4),* Special issue: Serving People with Psychiatric Disability at Risk for HIV/AIDS.

Susser, E., Valencia, E., & Torres, J. 1994. Sex, games, and videotapes: An HIV/prevention intervention for men who are homeless and have mental illness. *Psychosocial Rehabilitation Journal 17(4):* 31–40.

Toffler, A. 1970. *Future Shock.* New York: Random House.

2

Program Announcements and Requests for Applications
Signals to the Field

Willo Pequegnat

Program Announcements (PAs) and Requests for Applications (RFAs) can be important signals to the research community that an area is a major research initiative of the Institute. Often this means that budget requests have been built into future years to support research in this area. While an Institute will always accept an investigator-initiated research application, one that relates to an area where there is a paucity of work can be important in balancing a research portfolio. While the quality of the scientific review and priority score will be the most critical aspect of receiving funding, under the criteria for making an award, the program is given some latitude to consider priority of the research area.

NIMH has Program Announcements in the area of HIV infection and AIDS, some in collaboration with other NIH Institutes and the Public Health Service. Synopses of the Program Announcements are provided below for your information. (See Table 1 for a listing.)[1] In addition, information is provided on supplements for minority investigators.

Research is supported through approximately fifteen extramural research mechanisms, such as research project grants, Research Scientist Development Awards, institutional and individual research training grants, multidisciplinary AIDS research centers, and the Intramural Research Program (IRP).

---

[1] To receive a set of Program Announcements write to the Office on AIDS, NIMH, Parklawn Building, Room 10-75, 5600 Fishers Lane, Rockville, MD 20857, or call 301-443-7281.

Table 1. Program Announcements–AIDS Expedited Receipt Deadlines[a]

Brain, immune system, and behavioral and neurological aspects of Human Immunodeficiency Virus infection

Central nervous system effects of Human Immunodeficiency Virus infection: Neurobiological, neurovirological, and neurobehavioral studies

Neuro-AIDS: HIV-1 infection and the nervous system

Research on behavior change and prevention strategies to reduce transmission of Human Immunodeficiency Virus (HIV)

Determinants of effective HIV counseling

Measurement, course, and treatment of HIV-related mental disorders

Research on severely mentally ill persons at risk of or with HIV infections

Children with HIV infection and AIDS

Research Training

National Research Service Awards (NRSA) for institution research training grants in Human Immunodeficiency Virus (HIV) Infection and Acquired Immunodeficiency Syndrome (AIDS)[b]

National Research Service Awards (NRSA)[b] for research training for individual fellows in Human Immunodeficiency Virus (HIV) Infection Acquired Immunodeficiency Syndrome (AIDS)[c]

[a] The AIDS expedited review dates are January 2, May 1, and September 1.
[b] The submission date for NRSA Institutional applications is only once a year on May 10.
[c] The receipt dates for NRSA Individual grants (fellowships) are January 10, May 10, and September 10.

Brain, Immune System, and Behavioral and Neurological Aspects of Human Immunodeficiency Virus Infection

A major effect of HIV is to attack components of the immune system and leave the body vulnerable to a wide range of opportunistic infections. Scientific research has suggested that immune function can be influenced by neurological and psychological factors. The brain is hypothesized to be the organ through which environmental and psychological factors modify immune function. Research is needed to understand the regulation of immune responses by behavioral processes operating through the central nervous system (CNS) and endocrine systems. Studies in humans and animals are also needed to examine the interactions among these systems and to assess the role of repeated stressful events on immune function. Since the HIV virus has been shown to invade the CNS, basic neuroimmunological studies are needed to understand the etiology and pathology of HIV infection of the brain and the neurological and psychiatric sequelae of such infections. Work that addresses the CNS effects of HIV and AIDS Dementia Complex (ADC) is encouraged. Research that assesses neuropsychological and cognitive impairment in seropositive individuals using a standard core battery will be supported.[2] In addition, NIMH proposes to increase research on the incidence, prevalence, and natural history of HIV infection as part of this initiative.

Central Nervous System Effects of Human Immunodeficiency Virus Infection: Neurobiological, Neurovirological, and Neurobehavioral Studies

Early in the history of the AIDS epidemic, it was thought that the CNS disability seen in AIDS patients was a result of opportunistic infections on lymphomas. In fact, AIDS Dementia Complex (ADC), which is comprised of cognitive, motoric, and affective components, is now thought to be caused directly by HIV infection of the brain. In a short period of time, therefore, the relevance of neuroscience and the importance of the CNS in understanding AIDS have become apparent. Data clearly demonstrate HIV, the viral agent etiological for AIDS, enters the central nervous system (CNS) early in the course of this infection. Clinical observations have demonstrated that CNS impairment is common by the time the infection has advanced to AIDS. Based on these observations, the CDC case definition of AIDS was altered to include AIDS Dementia Complex (ADC) as sufficient for the diagnosis of AIDS in seropositive individuals without opportunistic infections or Kaposi's sarcoma lesions. This study proposes to examine the impact of HIV on the CNS from route of infection to neurobehavioral dysfunction and strategies to prevent the negative consequences of HIV.

Neuro-AIDS: HIV-1 Infection and the Nervous System

Neurological abnormalities and associated psychomotor and neurodevelopmental problems may be the first presenting symptoms of AIDS. Many advanced AIDS patients exhibit neurological dysfunction, and as many as 90 percent of the cases may demonstrate neuropathological changes at autopsy. It appears that the AIDS virus enters and affects the nervous system by way of macrophage infection and release of neurotoxic cytokines. In primary neuro-AIDS, involvement of every level of the central and peripheral nervous system (PNS) has been reported: dementia, meningitis, encephalitis, encephalopathy, myelopathy, peripheral neuropathy, and polymyositis. Myopathies, neuropathies, and other neurological side effects of current treatment are also known. Management and treatment of neurological complications of opportunistic infection and HIV-related malignancies remain a significant challenge. This PA is intended to motivate individual neuroscientists to become scientifically integrated in partnership with investigators supported by other NIH Institutes. Studies of HIV-1 infection of the CNS and subsequent neuro-AIDS complications in adults and children are encouraged as well as studies of AIDS-associated disorders of the PNS and resulting dysfunctions and abnormalities and epidemiological studies of neuro-AIDS, to name only a few.

---

[2] NIMH has developed a recommended battery for early detection of cognitive problems in asymptomatic seropositive persons (Butters *et al.,* 1990).

Research on Behavior Change and Prevention Strategies to Reduce Transmission of Human Immunodeficiency Virus

The major objective of the research supported under this initiative is to identify effective ways to prevent and foster changes in behaviors that place persons at high risk for infection by the HIV virus (e.g., high-risk sexual practices, intravenous drug use, etc.). Current research indicates that the acquisition of knowledge through educational materials, while necessary, is not sufficient to produce change in many individuals who participate in high-risk behaviors. Relevant research is encouraged to improve knowledge and understanding of the distribution of risk behaviors and to determine which factors or combination of factors are most successful in producing and sustaining behavior change, and under what conditions. Study populations or target groups should be those most likely to be engaging in high-risk behaviors.

Determinants of Effective HIV Counseling

The primary objective is to understand the determinants of effectively using HIV serotesting and counseling as preventive interventions with drug abusers, their sexual partners, and others at risk for HIV infection. Determinants of negative behavioral outcomes should also be examined. Risk behavior and other variables should be theoretically based. Although prospective studies are encouraged, retrospective studies that examine outcome, process, and social context variables of programs with documented successful impact on risk would be considered.

Children with HIV Infection and AIDS

This Program Announcement is intended to highlight specific areas with respect to infants and children with HIV infection and AIDS and their families and caregivers. Children are among the growing number of persons who are infected HIV. AIDS is a leading cause of death among children between the ages of 1 and 4. Infants and children are infected with HIV by acquiring it from their mothers, from contaminated blood products or blood transfusions, or through sexual abuse. The CNS complications of AIDS have a different natural course in infants and young children than in adults; this may be attributable to the differing impact of the virus on a developing and plastic nervous system. It is imperative that the role of HIV in the CNS be understood more fully so that remedial procedures may be used to avert its devastating effects. A major action of the HIV is to attack components of the immune system and make the infant and child vulnerable to a host of opportunistic infections, bacterial infections, and pulmonary diseases. Research is needed to understand the regulation of immune responses by the CNS and endocrine system. Because infants and children are not always able to provide competent diagnostic information and other informants (e.g., parents, foster care providers, clinical interviewers, etc.) may not provide reliable or complete information, alternative methods of assessment are needed. In addition to better assessment measures, there is a need for outcome measures that are realistic in evaluating the efficacy of different interventions on different domains of functioning for infants and children and their families. In addition to manifesting clinical neurological problems, infants and children with HIV infection and AIDS can manifest concomitant psychiatric and behavioral disorders, but there is little existing research on these issues. The spectrum of psychopathological and neuropsychological manifestations of HIV infection and the course of these manifestations have not been described. Studies are needed of the risk factors related to the progression of HIV and the particular mental disorders that are experienced by infants and children that may be different from adults. Various therapies and psychosocial interventions appear promising for symptomatic children; studies are needed to evaluate the efficacy of these interventions.

Research on Severely Mentally Ill Persons at Risk of or with HIV Infection

This Program Announcement is designed to encourage investigator-initiated research on the risk of HIV infections in severely mentally ill persons and on the management of seropositivity in those with severe mental illness. Some of the issues to be addressed are the determination of the prevalence of HIV infections among severely mentally ill persons, including those who are homeless or reside in transient quarters. An assessment needs to be made about the nature and extent of sexual behaviors among the severely mentally ill that place them at risk of developing HIV infections as well as other risk behaviors that put them at risk of developing STDs. Some methods of education and behavior change that may be effective in reducing behaviors that place severely mentally ill at risk for HIV infection need to be developed and tested. Research on mental health service needs and provision of mental health services to persons with HIV infection who are mentally ill need to be undertaken.

Measurement, Course, and Treatment of HIV-Related Mental Disorders

The purpose of this Program Announcement is to stimulate clinical and epidemiological research in three major areas. First, studies are solicited that are directed at the measurement of HIV-related mental disorders by adapting or using existing neuropsychological, psychiatric, and psychosocial measurement instruments with good psychometric properties to assess the effects of HIV infection at different stages of the illness. In addition, studies that lead to the development of new instruments and techniques uniquely suited to HIV-related changes in mental status are sought. Next, studies that relate to the nature and course of the disease, which can range from identifying the incidence and prevalence of mental disorders in HIV infection and AIDS to assessing the relationship of mental disorder manifestations of HIV illness to other manifestations of HIV illness, are sought. Finally, this Program Announcement seeks to promote research that involves clinical treatment and prevention clinical trials for HIV-related mental disorders. This provides support for research focused on the HIV infection among the severely mentally ill as well as research on mental health services for HIV-infected individuals who develop HIV-related mental disorders.

National Research Service Awards for Institutional Research Training Grants in Human Immunodeficiency Virus Infection

The gravity and rising prevalence of HIV disease has prompted intensive scientific research spanning levels of inquiry ranging from molecular biology to the study of social and institutional behavior. Reflecting that range, current scientific efforts are notable for multidisciplinary approaches to the myriad of scientific problems associated with HIV infection and its impact on society. This approach has successfully yielded a great deal of information about the disease in a short time, but important dimensions of the disease remain unknown. Therefore, not only is there a need for increased research, but there is also an increasing need for well-trained researchers with a multidisciplinary perspective that characterizes research on this extraordinarily complex disease. The objective of this Program Announcement is to establish appropriate research training programs for both young and developing scientists as well as experienced investigators. Special areas of interest include: (1) psychosocial, prevention, and behavior change; (2) brain, immune system, and behavioral aspects of HIV infection; (3) central nervous system (CNS) effects of HIV infection; (4) mental health services research concerning persons with HIV infection and AIDS; and (5) clinical and epidemiologic research in the measurement, course, treatment, and prevention of HIV-related mental disorders.

National Research Service Awards for Research Training for Individual Fellows in Human Immunodeficiency Virus Infection

In addition to Institutional Research Training Grants (described above), there is also support provided to individual fellows to develop projects in the same areas of interest.

Small Business Innovation Research (SBIR)

The Small Business Innovation Development Act, P.L. 97-219 amended by P.L. 99-443, requires the agencies of PHS and certain other federal agencies reserve a specified amount of their extramural research and development (R&D) budgets for a Small Business Innovation Research (SBIR) Program. The legislation is intended to: (1) stimulate technological innovation, (2) use small business to meet federal research and development needs, (3) increase private sector commercialization of innovations derived from federal research and development, and (4) foster and encourage participation by minority and disadvantaged persons in technological innovation. The SBIR consists of three phases. The objective of phase I is to establish the technical merit and feasibility of the proposed research or R&D efforts and to determine the quality of performance of the small business awardee organization prior to providing further federal support. The objective of phase II is to continue the research or R&D efforts initiated in Phase I. Funding will be based on the results of Phase I and the scientific and technical merit of the Phase II application. The objective of Phase III is for the small business to pursue with non-federal funds the commercialization of the results of the research or R&D funded in Phases I and II.

Guidelines for Supplements for Underrepresented Minorities in Biomedical and Behavioral Research[3]

This provides for funding through administrative supplements to currently reviewed and funded grants to support minority scientists and students. The purpose is to attract and encourage minority individuals to

---

[3] This Program Announcement can be obtained from Delores L. Parron, Ph.D., Associate Director for Special Populations, NIMH, 5600 Fishers Lane, Room 17C-14, Rockville, MD 20857; 301-443-2847.

pursue research careers. The proposed research experience must be an integral part of the approved parent grant that has been peer-reviewed. Therefore, the decision to provide supplemental funding to the minority investigator can be made administratively in weeks rather than months.

You must find a funded Principal Investigator (PI) who is willing to be your mentor and help you to develop a small study that is derivative from the parent grant. The PI should submit a cover letter requesting the supplemental funds directly to the relevant Institute. You should also include: (1) a completed face page from PHS Grant Application Form 398 with the title and grant number of the parent grant and a statement that specifies which type of supplement (e.g., minority undergraduate student, minority graduate student, etc.) is being requested; (2) a brief (3- to 4-page) description prepared by the PI of the parent grant of the proposed research experience, how it will expand and foster the independent research capabilities of the minority individual, and how it relates to the research objectives of the parent grant; (3) a statement from the minority individual outlining his/her research objectives and career goals; (4) Social Security number and biographical sketch of the minority individual that includes evidence of scientific achievement; (5) a proposed budget entered on budget pages from the PHS Grant Application Form 398, related to the percent effort (where appropriate) for the research experience on the first year of the supplement and future years; (6) documentation, if applicable, that the proposed research experience was approved by the animal welfare committee or human subjects institutional review board of the grantee institution; and (7) a copy of an official transcript if the minority candidate is a student.

The request must be signed by the minority individual, the PI, and the appropriate institutional business official. If the minority individual is an employee of another institution, the request also must be accompanied by an appropriately signed letter from the institution of the minority individual indicating that participation at the stated level of effort is approved. If any of the research is to be conducted at a site other than the grantee institution, an appropriately signed letter from the institution where the research is to be conducted must also be submitted.

How Do You Find Out about Program Announcements?[4]

The National Institutes of Health (NIH) publishes the *NIH Guide to Grants and Contracts,* which serves as an early warning system for new research program initiatives across federal agencies. Information about research contracts are published in the *Commerce Clearinghouse Daily.* Your university research grant office should subscribe to both of these publications as well as have other information that will allow you to keep abreast of research opportunities in your area. In addition, you can call program staff at NIMH to discuss their evaluation of current and future program initiatives.

Improving Your Chances to Be Funded

A Program Announcement is a signal to the field from NIMH that this is an important research initiative. Your application will be reviewed by the standing Internal Review Group (IRG), which has diverse expertise. Funding is based on the percentile that your application receives and how your application complements the priority areas of the NIMH research program. Your chances of being funded if you are in the fundable range may be slightly improved if your application is in a priority area.

---

[4] See "Selecting Issues and Hypotheses for a Research Proposal" by Manson, this volume, on techniques for anticipating federal research initiatives.

Another mechanism that may improve your chance of being funded is responding to a Request for Applications (RFA). This is an even stronger signal to the field that this is a priority area because there is a designated amount of money attached to this initiative. A Special Review Committee (SRC), rather than the regular IRG, will review your application. This has three distinct advantages: (1) a designated amount of money, (2) the SRC will only have reviewers tailored to the specific expertise of the IRG, and (3) the grants will be funded on the basis of its percentile, but there may be more latitude.

An RFA may be a cooperative agreement. If you are committed to conducting the study that you have designed, you may not wish to submit a proposal in response to this RFA even if it is in your area.[5] First, such a mechanism allows NIMH staff to play a major role in the design of the final protocol. Next, your research application is an opportunity for you to demonstrate that you have competent research skills, the necessary resources and environment, and access to research subjects. If funded, you will become part of a clinical trial implementing a standard protocol. This process ensures high visibility for your work as a PI but not the usual independence in conducting a study associated with that role.

Important Categories in a Program Announcement

Each Program Announcement will have many of the same features; however, different kinds of Announcements may have slightly different sections. The front page of the Program Announcement will have: (1) the name of the Program Announcement, (2) the sponsoring Institute(s), and (3) the authority under which it is issued.

Purpose of Program Announcement

This is a brief statement about the problem that the Program Announcement is designed to address and the goals of the program.

Background to the Program Announcement

This provides the historical background for the problem.

Areas of Interest

This section enumerates some of the potential research topics. These are only examples, and you should not feel limited by the topics.

Eligibility to Apply

This lists the types of organizations and institutions that can apply. For example, foreign institutions are eligible on some PAs or RFAs but not others.

Inclusion of Minorities and Women in Study Populations

Public Health Service (PHS) policy requires that minorities and women be included in research populations. This is a specific criterion that will be discussed during the scientific review and in your summary

---

[5] See "Developing a Budget and Financial Justification" by Mucha, this volume, which describes the U01 and U10 cooperative agreements.

Table 2. Expedited Receipt and Review Schedule for AIDS Applications			
Receipt Dates	**Scientific Review**	**Council Review**	**Earliest Award**
January 2	Feb/March	May/June	June
May 1	June/July	Sept/Oct	Sept 30
September 1	Oct/Nov	Jan/Feb	Feb

statement. If you do not include minorities or women in your study, be specific about the reason so that the IRG can consider it as part of its scientific review.[6]

AIDS IRB Guidelines

Because AIDS grants have an expedited review, they cannot be assigned for peer review until IRB approval is obtained.

Review Procedures and Criteria

This section enumerates the review procedures that will be used to ensure that you receive a fair and competent review of your research application. In addition, the review criteria that will be used by the IRG are stated. These are important because the review committee will use these criteria in receiving your research application.

Award Criteria

Ordinarily, grants are funded in order of percentile ranking; however, if your grant addresses a high priority area or meets other criteria specified in this section, your chances may be slightly improved.

Receipt and Review Schedule

AIDS is on an expedited receipt and review schedule, which means it has different receipt dates and a more rapid referral process. Congress requires that your grant is referred, reviewed, and a funding decision made within six months. This section lists the specific receipt dates, the months during which the IRG will probably review, the dates of the Council, and finally the earliest date that you could receive funding. (See also Table 2.)

Application Submission Instructions

This section provides information on where to obtain the PHS 398 application package and the number of copies to send to the appropriate address.

[6] See the instructions in the PHS Form 398 (Rev. 9/91), Appendix C (this volume), for guidelines on gender and minority inclusion in proposed studies.

Mechanisms of Support

This lists the kinds of mechanisms that can be used under this announcement (e.g., R01, R03, R29). In some instances, it may not be possible to submit a small grant, a program project, or some other mechanism of support.[7]

Terms and Conditions of Support

This section discusses direct costs associated with the cost of the actual project and the allowable indirect costs of the institution. It also discusses the amount of time for which support can be made for this project.

Further Information

These are the staff contacts from sponsoring Institutes who most likely prepared the announcement. They are therefore interested in receiving good applications and can provide excellent technical assistance.

Referral to an Initial Review Group (IRG)

When you apply in response to a specific Program Announcement, put its number and title in the Block 2 on the face page of the PHS 398 and on the container used to mail the application and check the YES box. This can be important because it may determine where your application is referred for review.

The title of your research application and abstract are also critical in the process referral and will be read by more people than any other part of your proposal. If you want your application referred to NIMH, be sure to relate your project to issues in mental health. In addition, you can include a cover letter indicating the NIMH staff person with whom you worked in developing your research application. Finally, you should ask the program person with whom you worked to put in a form requesting that your application be referred to NIMH.

Appendix: Department of Health and Human Services Public Health Service, National Institutes of Health, National Institute of Mental Health (May 1994)

The National Institute of Mental Health periodically issues a list of current Program Announcements. Single copies of the Announcements may be requested from Anne Cooley, Division of Extramural Activities, NIMH, Parklawn Building, Room 9C-04, 5600 Fishers Lane, Rockville, Maryland 20857. The telephone number is 301-443-4673.

Research and Research Career Development	Date Issued
Extramural Research Support Programs	6/94 (rev.)
Prevention Intervention Research Centers	2/94 (rev.)

---

[7] See "Selecting the Appropriate Research Mechanism" by Friedenberg *et al.*, this volume.

First Independent Research Support and Transition (FIRST) Award (R29)	9/93 (rev.)
Public-Academic Liaison (PAL) for Research on Serious Mental Disorders	9/88
Studies of Suicide and Suicidal Behavior	1/94 (rev.)
Minority Institutions Research Development Program	4/89
Small Business Innovation Research (SBIR) (with NIH)	1/94 (rev.)
Behavioral and Neural Approaches to Cognition in Mental Health and Mental Disorders, PA-91-03	10/90
Rapid Assessment Post-Impact of Disaster (RAPID), PA-91-04	9/90
Small Grant Program (with NIAA and NIDA) (RO3) PA-91-08	10/90 (rev.)
Investigations into Methods that Replace or Reduce Vertebrate Animals Used in Research or Lessen Their Pain or Distress (with NIAAA, NIDA, NIH), PA-91-20	1/91
Psychopathology and Mental Retardation, PA-91-37	2/91 (rev.)
Clinical Mental Health Academic Award (K07), PA-91-38	3/91
Child and Adolescent Mental Health Service System Research Demonstration Grants, PA-91-40	4/91
Specialized Mental Health Clinical Research Centers, General Mental Health Clinical Research Centers, PA-91-43	4/91 (rev.)
Implementation for the National Plan for Research on Child and Adolescent Mental Disorders, PA-91-46	4/91
Research on Mental Disorders in Rural Populations PA-91-52	5/94 (rev.)
Combined Psychosocial and Pharmacologic Treatments Research, PA-91-54	4/91
Research on Hospitalization of Adolescents for Mental Disorders, PA-91-58	4/91
Mental Health Research on Homeless Persons, PA-91-68	2/94 (rev.)
Research on Managed Health Care, PA-91-71	6/91
Research on Disabilities and Rehabilitation Services for Persons with Severe Mental Disorders, PA-91-74	7/91
Anorexia Nervosa and Bulimia Nervosa: Basic Brain Behavioral and Clinical Studies, PA-91-79	6/91
Multi-Institutional Collaborative Research Project, (R10) PA-91-81	7/91

Special Issues in Women's Mental Health Over the Life Cycle, PA-91-100   9/91

Research Scientist Development Award (K02), PA-91-101   9/91 (rev.)

Research Scientist Award (K05), PA-91-102   9/91 (rev.)

Research on Law and Mental Health, PA-92-01   9/91

Research on Victims of Traumatic Stress, PA-92-02   9/91

Research on Perpetrators of Violence, PA-92-03   9/91

Research Grants on Neural Systems and Mental, Neurological and Aging Disorders, PA-92-07   7/91

Psychotherapeutic Drug Discovery and Development Program, PA-92-15   9/91

Centers for Research on Mental Health Services for Children and Adolescents, PA-92-20   11/91

Depression in Late Life, PA-92-44   2/92

Implementation of Caring for People with Severe Mental Disorders: A National Plan of Research to Improve Services, PA-92-65   4/92

Social Work Research Development Centers, PA-92-78   4/92

Centers for Research on Services for People with Severe Mental Disorders, PA-92-94   6/92

Scientist Development Award for Clinicians (K20), PA-92-98 (with NIDA and NIAAA)   8/92 (rev.)

Scientist Development Award (K21), PA-92-99 (with NIDA and NIAAA)   8/92 (rev.)

Research on Mental Health Services in the General Health Care Sector, PA-92-103   9/92

Women's Health Over the Lifecourse: Social and Behavioral Aspects, PA-92-105 (with NIA and NICHD)   9/92

Minority Mental Health Research Centers, PA-92-122   9/92

Child and Adolescent Development and Psychopathology Research Centers (CADPRC), PA-93-02   5/93

Research Infrastructure Support Program (RISP) PA-93-03   9/92

Neural, Endocrine, Immune, and Viral Interactions, Behavior, and Mental Health, PA-93-009	10/92
Centers for AIDS Research Core Grant Support (CFAR CSG), (with NIAID), A1-93-14	7/93
American Indian, Alaska Native, and Native Hawaiian Mental Health Research, PA-93-53	2/93
Comparative Approaches to Brain and Behavior, PA-93-57	2/93
Small Grant Program (NIH)	3/93 (rev.)
Small Business Innovation Research (SBIR) (with NIH)	1/94 (rev.)
Investigator-Initiated Interactive Research Project Grants (multi-institutional), PA-93-78	4/93
The Human Brain Project: Phase I Feasibility Studies, PA-93-068	4/93
Research on Emergency Mental Health Services for Children and Adolescents, PA-93-075	5/93
Determinants of Effective HIV Counseling (with NIDA), PA-93-080	4/93
Research on Integrating Mental Health and Related Services for Persons with Severe Mental Disorders PA-93-088	5/93
Experimental/Developmental Grants (R21) for Psychosocial Treatment Research, PA-93-093	5/93
Research on Mental Health Economics, PA-94-018	12/93
Academic Research Enhancement Award (AREA)	1/94
Minority Dissertation Research Grants in Mental Health, PAR-94-053	4/94
Basic Research in Emotion (with NIH), PA-94-059	1/94
Research on Methods, Measurement and Statistical Analysis in Mental Health Research, PA-94-060	4/94
Dissertation Research Grants in: Child and Adolescent Developmental Psychopathology, HIV/AIDS Research, Mental Health Services Research, PAR-94-063	4/94
Research Program on Prescription Drug Use, Abuse and Diversion (with NIDA), PA-94-070	6/94

Research Training

Minority Access to Research Careers (MARC)

Honors Undergraduate Research Training Grants	3/87 (rev.)
Faculty Fellowship Awards	3/87 (rev.)

National Research Service Awards (with NIAAA and NIDA)

Individual Fellowships

Predoctoral (F31), PAR-93-040	4/94 (rev.)
Postdoctoral (F32), PA-94-055	4/94 (rev.)
Institutional Training Grants (T32), PA-92-31	1/92 (rev.)
National Research Service Awards for Predoctoral *Individual* M.D./Ph.D. Fellows (F30)	3/89
Short-Term *Institutional* National Research Service Awards (T35), PA-92-92	9/92
NRSA *Institutional* Training Grants for AIDS (with NIAID), PA-93-087	5/93
Academic Research Enhancement Award (AREA)	1/94
Supplements to Promote Reentry into Biomedical and Biobehavioral Research Careers, PA-94-040	3/94

Other

Awards for Mental Health Services to Cuban Entrants	10/83

Subject to availability of funds and to periodical modification of areas supported, applications for new research and research career development grants will be accepted by NIMH under the receipt dates of February 1, June 1, and October 1. (Receipt dates for competing renewal and competing supplemental research and research career development applications are March 1, July 1, and November 1.) The receipt dates for individual research fellowships are January 10, May 10, and September 10; institutional NRSA research training grant applications are accepted only on May 10.

Receipt dates for Small Business Innovation Research applications are April 15, August 15, and December 15.

Receipt dates for all unsolicited new and competing renewal AIDS research grant applications are January 2, May 1, and September 1 of each year.

Reference

Butters, N., Grant, I., Haxby, J., Judd, L. L., Martin, A., McClelland, J., Pequegnat, W., Schacter, D., & Stover, E. 1990. Assessment of AIDS-related cognitive changes: Recommendations of the NIMH Workshop on Neuropsychological Assessment Approaches. *Journal of Clinical and Experimental Neuropsychological Assessment Approaches 12:* 963–978.

3

Grantsmanship
A View from Inside and Out

Raymond P. Lorion

In this chapter, I share some thoughts about the preparation and submission of an application for research funding. My comments are based on a variety of experiences relating to "grantsmanship," the strategies and perspectives associated with experienced (and successful) applicants for funding. Over the past decade, I have served as a Visiting Scientist to the National Institute of Mental Health, an Acting Associate Administrator and policy and program consultant to many parts of the Alcohol, Drug Abuse, and Mental Health Administration (ADAMHA); an *ad hoc* reviewer and member of a peer review panel; and an applicant for training, research, and program development funds. Through these experiences, I have achieved some understanding of the process underlying the formation of funding policies and the attitudes, perspectives, and strategies of successful applicants.

As an overarching principle, it is important to appreciate that funding opportunities represent both political and scientific processes. Program Announcements (Requests For Applications [RFAs] or Requests For Proposals [RFPs]) are intended to reflect the current state of science and encourage increases in its breadth and depth.[1] By selectively encouraging systematic investigations in promising areas, federal agencies seek to increase our understanding of known mechanisms and to identify as yet unknown contributors to emotional and behavioral functioning.

Funding limitations necessitate the establishment of priorities. The process by which priorities are set, promising issues identified, and "cutting edge" opportunities selected involves a merging of scientific knowledge and systematic debate and input from multiple sources. The latter, obviously, represents a "political" process in the sense that credible scientists differ in their estimations of the heuristic potential of areas of inquiry. These divergent views are presented and debated, and decisions are made following the planful analysis of relevant bodies of information. Understanding the bases used to arrive at such decisions is an important element of grantsmanship. In effect, careful analysis of the state of knowledge

[1] Editors' note: See "Program Announcements and Requests for Applications: Signals to the Field" by Pequegnat, this volume.

39

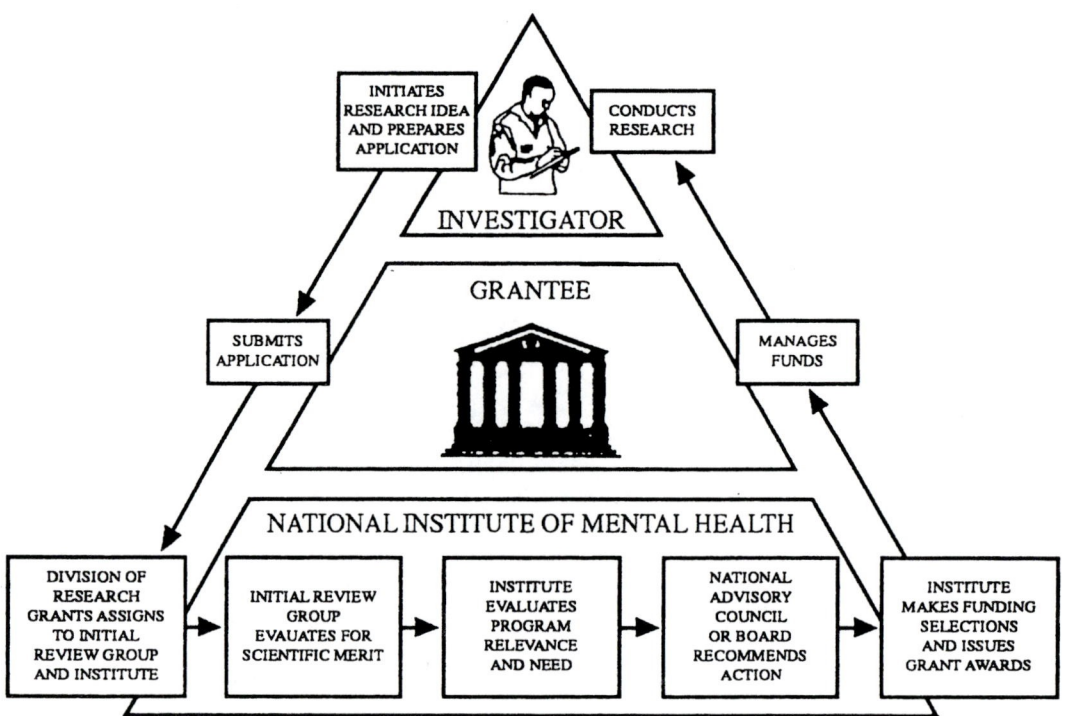

Figure 1. The grant process.

of a field contributes to the establishment of priorities. That same level of analysis will subsequently be applied in the review of applications and decisions related to funding levels.

A recent and highly visible research initiative, "Decade of the Brain," evolved from this combined scientific and political process.[2] While some may argue that too much emphasis will be placed on biological processes and that some segments of the mental health research community were overly influential, close examination of the decision-making process reveals that the initiative reflects the momentum of the scientific process and of discovery. The initiative and the funding priorities associated with it reflect the enthusiasm, encouragement, and support for a body of research whose conduct is producing vast increments in our understanding of emotional and behavioral health.

Funding priorities among Institutes are also political in the sense that they reflect a balance among scientific and theoretical emphases, social concerns, and public health issues. In HIV research, for example, political concerns, namely the public's concern about AIDS, are driving the science to focus its energies and its resources on this significant threat to human health. Independent of how sophisticated and advanced the scientific knowledge base is, the public's demand for prevention and treatment efforts must be vigorously pursued on a national basis. In effect, what is currently known must be applied at the same time that priority is given to expanding that knowledge base. These views, in turn, have been translated into NIMH's research opportunities in HIV research.

Finally, it is important to recognize the human element in the grant review process. Submission of an application for funding is, in fact, a communication between one scientist and other knowledgeable

[2] Editors' note: The Office of AIDS Programs, NIMH prepared a document entitled "AIDS Research: An NIMH Blueprint for the Second Decade," which lays out research initiatives for the next ten years.

scientists. Not unlike other communications, the elements of respect, openness, acceptance, and compromise are important components of the dialogue. It is also important to appreciate the diversity of people involved in the grant process (e.g., NIMH staff, current grantees, and potential members of review group). Each of these groups has a commitment to achieving the demanding balance between maximizing each applicant's competitiveness for funding and maximizing the scientific and public health benefits of funding decisions. Over time, it has become increasingly clear that the process rarely involves "good guys" and "bad guys." Rather, it involves many people spending long hours making difficult decisions.

On the human side, it is valuable to understand that the NIMH staff exist not only to administer research programs, but also to nurture the development of the scientists supported by such programs. For the staff, every funded grantee is a client to be served and encouraged to meet the scientific promises of the existing application and to submit additional highly competitive applications. NIMH staff are as invested in the careers of the investigators as are the investigators themselves. Thus, staff will assist potential applicants to develop an application. If the proposal is approved, they are available to help accomplish the specific aims of the research. If the application is not approved, the NIMH staff assist the applicant in understanding what the summary statement means and in providing advice about resubmission.[3]

The following suggestions are culled from my personal experience with the grant process, both as a program person within the system and as an investigator outside the system. Figure 1 provides a graphic representation of the grant process.

Presubmission Consultation

Presubmission consultation, especially with NIMH staff, is a very important first step for applicants. This is particularly true for a project that may be methodologically innovative or outside the mainstream of HIV research. If you have an idea, call someone at NIMH and give them a brief description of your proposal.[4] The staff knows what is being funded and can give you an idea of how your proposal would fit into the existing grant portfolio. Staff know who received funding recently and whose research has not yet appeared in the literature. This information may provide you with valuable resources for consultation, expand the comprehensiveness of your literature review, or identify alternative research strategies. Having attended recent application reviews, the staff can provide an informed estimate of the idea's competitiveness and proximity to the cutting edge.

Thus, I encourage you to ask the staff for the names of others who are doing similar research that you can contact. You may consider adding these researchers as consultants to your application. Call your fellow researchers and talk to them about your proposal. Find out what mistakes they may have made and concerns they have about this area of research. Understand that many experienced and active researchers receive such requests frequently and view their response as part of our scientific responsibility.

Develop a Prospectus

The second step in the application process is to develop a 3- to 5-page prospectus in which you describe the two or three major questions that you want to ask. This will help the staff link your proposal to other

---

[3] Editors' note: See "Reading between the Lines of Your Summary Statement" by Lyman, this volume.

[4] Editors' note: If you are responding to a Program Announcement, look under the section in the back of the PA for the names of the people to contact for more information.

projects being funded. It should be succinct and lay out the questions to be asked, the methodology to be employed, the measures that exist and those that need to be developed, and the procedures that are proposed. If possible, a budget and time frame would be useful in making an initial evaluation. Your prospectus does not require a detailed literature review.

Members of the Review Committee

Ask the NIMH staff for the names of the members of the review committee who will review your research application.[5] Staff cannot tell you who the primary, secondary, and tertiary reviewers will be because the assignments are confidential and are the responsibility of the Scientific Review Administrator (SRA) in the Division of Extramural Activities (DEA), NIMH.[6] You will need to do your homework and find out which member has expertise that is relevant to your proposal. For example, your proposal may require teacher ratings, and a member of the committee has developed a teacher rating scale. You do not need to use that person's scale, but you should mention it in order to demonstrate awareness of the range of measures available. As reviewers, we do not expect that only our work will be cited or our methodologies used. We do, however, expect that the applicant be aware of alternative approaches and provide a scientific rationale for procedures selected and procedures rejected.

If there is not a standing review committee, assess who is making the major contributions to the journals on the topic of your research. Ask staff if there are any recent NIMH reviews or monographs related to your topic. Some of the most up-to-date, important scientific reports are not available in the journals but are found in publications prepared by the Institutes. Frequently, the same experts that the Institute invited to speak at its conferences or prepare a chapter in a monograph will be those asked to review grants.

Submit Comments on First Draft of Your Research Application

The draft of your proposal should be completed no later than six weeks prior to the submission date. This will permit you to receive comments from several different audiences. The most obvious is to have someone who currently has a grant in the same area read your proposal. However, you need to be sure that person is not a current member of a group that might review your grant after it is submitted. If so, do not forward your draft, because that person would then be disqualified as a reviewer of your proposal. Similarly, if you feel the person would make a good *ad hoc* reviewer for your proposal, do not send it to him or her.

You should also show your proposal to someone who is in another discipline or who is not a researcher. If that person can understand your proposal, then it will probably be clear to the reviewers. Ask the person to make notes about the assumptions with which he or she does not agree and parts of the grant that are not clear. These comments will help you identify where you may have left out part of your thought process that you take for granted but which may be required in order to understand the specific aims of your study.

[5] Editors' note: At NIMH, the review committee is called the Initial Review Group (IRG).

[6] Editors' note: Each research application is usually reviewed by three persons who have responsibility to read your proposal carefully. At the IRG meeting they provide a verbal review and a written report, which forms the basis of the summary statement, along with the discussion of your research application.

Link Past, Present, and Future Developments in the Field

All reviewers evaluate whether a potential grantee has a sense of the current state of the field. You should demonstrate that you know how your ideas flow from what has already been done and potentially could contribute new knowledge. Reviewers will assess whether you will be able to modify your study if your methodology does not work. One way of demonstrating this is by showing that you know what others have done and by specifying problems you might anticipate and how you might overcome them. This is particularly true when you are new to the grant-funding process. Reviewers do not expect that conducting your study is going to be problem free, but they do want a sense that you appreciate the difference between how research is proposed and how it actually may be conducted.

Consultants[7]

Assess areas where expertise is required to conduct your study and where your curriculum vitae (CV) does not demonstrate that expertise. If you are proposing complex statistical procedures and you are not experienced in the application and interpretation of structural modeling and multivariate analyses, for example, name a statistical consultant who can help you at critical points in the development of your study, and request a reasonable percentage time in the budget for this expertise.[8] If you are conducting epidemiological surveys to evaluate the needs prior to the intervention, request an expert in survey methods and field research. Recognize that the reviewers must evaluate whether you have a good question, are posing it in a way that can be answered, and have reflected, through your time table, budget, and procedures, the necessary experience and foresight to carry out the project. If this requires you to hire consultants, they should be named, if possible, and, if they are critical to the success of the study, their CV should be included in the research application.

Develop a Timeline

The basic rule of thumb in research is that everything takes longer than you think. For a reviewer, the issue is not how fast can you do a project, but whether you do it in a timeframe that is realistic to the research involved. If you state that you are going to hire and train staff and recruit all your subjects in three months, a reviewer will be skeptical unless you can give clear evidence that it is feasible. Piloting each of these components singly and in combination represents a convincing way to reduce that skepticism.

You should include in the proposal a timeline that indicates when your independent variable (intervention) will be implemented and when evaluation of your dependent variables (instruments) will occur. The timeline is important because it allows the reviewer to grasp quickly the design of your study. It also provides the reviewer with a sense of the measurement demand on each one of your data sources. For example, it will reveal whether you are asking teachers to provide 3½ hours of information on each pupil. This may be necessary in your view but unlikely to be accomplished in the reviewers' experience. Far too

---

[7] Editors' note: See "Developing a Résumé and Presenting a Staff" by Mitnick, this volume.

[8] Editors' note: 10% time is about 4 hours a week; it may be that it would be better to have the expert 1 day every other week or for 2 days at the beginning of the year and 2 weeks during the summer. Specify the time that is required to complete the tasks the consultant is requested to do for your project.

often, for example, I have reviewed proposals that recruit children throughout the year but ignore the fact that teachers may be unavailable to provide ratings during the summer months.

A timeline will also allow you to determine whether your staff will be adequate to cover all the assessments scheduled. This, in turn, may help you plan a more efficient sequence of evaluations for your project.

Budget

The budget should reflect a realistic evaluation of what resources are needed to conduct your study as designed. If a researcher states that interview sessions will be recorded and analyzed, a quick calculation reveals that there will be approximately 3,500 hours of raw tape. It takes 2–3 hours to do a content analysis of 1 hour of tape; it will take approximately 10,000 hours to analyze the tape, only 10% of which would be covered by the requested grant funds. Requesting a videotape machine and 1,000 hours of an undergraduate research assistant at $5 an hour would therefore be inadequate.

Ensuring Confidentiality[9]

Even though your research application has been approved by your local Institutional Review Board (IRB), reviewers will evaluate whether you have adequately guaranteed the confidentially of your research subjects. Reviewers are responsible for doing this independent review of your human subjects procedures, and in areas like drug abuse, criminal justice, conduct disorder, and AIDS, the reviewers spend time examining your safeguards for confidentiality. You should talk to your project officer about obtaining a Certificate of Confidentiality, which ensures confidentiality of your data after they are collected.[10]

Reviewers will also examine the procedures to be used for the control (i.e. non-intervention subjects) that are in need of service. Are your control subjects going to receive the intervention when the study is over, and, if so, how will you ensure that they know about this opportunity? What are your contingencies for handling a crisis situation during the study: Are you going to initiate an intervention for them, which will mean that they will be lost to the study? There may not be a clear answer to some of these questions, but you must demonstrate to the reviewers that you are aware of possible ethical dilemmas and that you have a procedure for handling them. In some cases, you may want to use an advisory group to oversee protection of your human subjects.

Anticipate Rejection

The reality of the grant process is that, generally, only one out of four applications may be approved and fewer still receive a priority score and percentile ranking that results in funding. You must therefore anticipate that you will not receive funding the first time that you submit your research application. If you have responded to a Program Announcement, you should consider submitting a revised research applica-

[9] Editors' note: See "Institutional Review Boards and Special Human Subject Issues in AIDS Research" by Rabkin, this volume.

[10] Editors' note: You can obtain a Certificate of Confidentiality by submitting a request to the Division of Extramural Activities (DEA), which conducts the reviews.

tion.[11] Your summary statement (pink sheet) may substantially contribute to improving your grant approval. For example, the reviewers may have raised questions about an analytical problem in your proposal that may suggest useful alternatives.

NIMH staff are permitted to attend the meeting where your grant is reviewed. They are not allowed to contribute to the review process, but they can take notes that can be shared with you after you have received the summary statement. For example, they can tell you whether the committee was interested in pursuing your proposal with some changes. Staff can provide clarification that will allow you to read between the lines of the summary statement (pink sheet).[12]

The Value of Persistence

Although the summary statement is a critique and not intended as a guideline for assured funding, if read carefully it can substantively contribute to your revisions. A resubmission that addresses substantive concerns may have a better chance of receiving a score in the fundable range than most first-time submissions. When you resubmit, begin with a summary of the reviewers' concerns and indicate where you address each concern in the revised proposal. This alerts the reviewers to look for the changes that potentially have improved your proposal. However, if you disagree with the reviewers' opinion, you are not required to make the change but you should state your rationale for not doing so.

If you review this handbook carefully and follow the suggestions that are made in each chapter, you will be well on your way to mastering the techniques of grantsmanship.

[11] Editors' note: If you have responded to an RFA, it may be a one-time submission date. In that case, you should talk to NIMH staff about an appropriate Program Announcement to which you might submit your revised research application.

[12] Editors' note: See "Reading between the Lines of Your Summary Statement" by Lyman, this volume.

4

The Review Process

Hugh Stamper

This is an overview of what happens to your grant application after you mail it to Bethesda. In describing the review process, I will begin at the point when your research application is received by the Division of Research Grants (DRG) at the National Institutes of Health (NIH), and follow through the sequence of events from referral to the NIMH to review by an Initial Review Group (IRG) and by the National Advisory Mental Health Council ("Council").

NIMH has a dedicated staff whose job is to ensure a proper review of your application. Nonetheless, because of the number of applications reviewed by the Institute each year and because aspects of an application can be overlooked or misinterpreted, it is important that you communicate with staff throughout the consideration of your application, particularly if you feel that the process is not proceeding properly.

Receipt and Referral: Assignment to Institute and IRG

After you send in your application, it arrives at a mailroom at the NIH and is one of approximately 35,000 to 40,000 applications received each year by DRG. (See Figure 1.)

Once an application has been received, DRG assigns it to an Institute and an IRG. The assignment is made by a referral officer using explicit written guidelines negotiated among the Institutes. Most applications on mental health are assigned to NIMH, but questions may appropriately arise if there is a potential overlap with the missions of other Institutes within the NIH.

If you feel that your application would be most appropriately assigned to the NIMH—and this is particularly true if you received advice from NIMH staff on your research project—you should state in a cover letter accompanying your application that you have been in contact with, say, Dr. Pequegnat of NIMH, that the research is particularly relevant to that Institute (be specific), and that you request assignment of your application accordingly. You may also request assignment to a particular program division within the Institute for grant monitoring if you wish. It is important to keep in mind that these

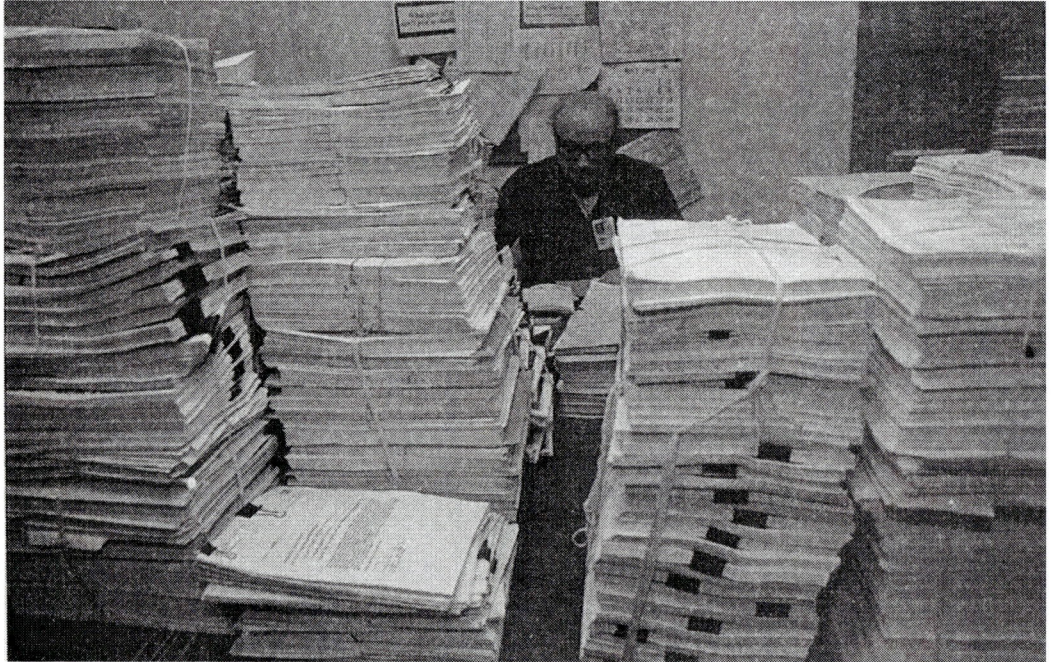

Figure 1. Referral officer making decisions about the review of AIDS research applications.

assignments are made on the basis of written guidelines; your "request" alone may not be sufficient to effect the assignment that you desire if the referral guidelines call for your application to go to another Institute.

The other part of your application's assignment, which is in some ways more important to you than the Institute or program to which it is sent, is to the IRG (also referred to at NIH as "study section").[1] It is extremely important that the IRG be appropriate to review your proposed research. Although there are referral guidelines for assigning applications to particular review committees, the appropriate committee is not always clear-cut, and judgment is often required on the part of the referral officer. Clearly, if you believe that one committee is more appropriate than another because of the required expertise, state that in the cover letter with your rationale. You may also suggest that certain areas of expertise are essential to ensure a sound scientific review (e.g., immunology, neuropsychology, etc.). This will alert referral personnel to your preference. If your request is not granted or you wish to question it, you should feel free to contact the referral officer.

As soon as the assignment is made, you are notified of the Institute assignment, the application's identification number, and the assigned IRG and the Scientific Review Administrator (SRA) responsible for that committee.

When an application is assigned to NIMH, the process from receipt of the application by the Institute through completion of the summary statement (i.e., the summary of the IRG proceedings) is the

[1] Editors' note: At the time that this book went to press, changes were occuring in the way that grants referred to NIMH may be assigned for review. Many will be reviewed by an NIH standing committee rather than an NIMH committee. This chapter, however, does describe how reviews are generally conducted.

responsibility of the Division of Extramural Activities (DEA).[2] During this period questions regarding your application should be with that division, whose staff include the SRAs (formerly known as Executive Secretaries) of the IRGs. After the summary statement has been prepared and released to the applicant, DEA is no longer the primary contact point, and you should seek the advice of the program staff in the division (or office) to which your research application was assigned.[3]

NIMH Review Procedures: The Role of DEA and the IRGs

If your application is assigned to NIMH, you will receive a letter from your SRA that will contain information including the date of the IRG meeting, additional materials that may be required to carry out the review, and a listing of the current members on the committee. You will also be informed about options if you have any concerns about how your application is being handled. If you have questions, you should immediately contact your SRA for assistance. You will also learn in this letter of the availability of the NIH appeals process. With the committee roster in hand, you should satisfy yourself that the committee is appropriate and able to give your application a full and fair scientific review. If you do not think that the expertise represented on the committee is adequate to evaluate your application, call your SRA and discuss your concerns. She or he may have overlooked something, or you may be unaware of something that the SRA can help you understand. Again, you may wish to discuss the possibility of outside opinions (*ad hoc* reviewers)[4] to increase the scope of expertise that is involved in the review of your application.

If necessary, you might also wish to contact the SRA to discuss sending additional materials to be considered during the review of your application. If, for example, you have pilot data that could strengthen your application and that you did not have at the time you sent in the application, you should ask the SRA whether it is still possible to send it. Of course, if it is too close to the meeting date, there may not be adequate time for it to be considered in the review. The SRA will make every effort to be accommodating in this regard so that all appropriate available information is included in the evaluation of your application.

Applications are generally mailed to the IRG members at least 5 weeks prior to the meeting. This is done so that reviewers have adequate time to fully study each application and prepare written comments that will ultimately be incorporated into the summary statement.

The IRG Meeting

The next step in the process is the review meeting itself, which takes place around a large table, with the chairperson and the SRA at the head of the table and program staff present and attending as observers. (See Figure 2.) Together, the chairperson of the IRG and the SRA monitor the review of each application not only from a scientific standpoint, but also to ensure that review criteria are appropriately applied,

---

[2] The address is DEA, Parklawn Building, Room 9-105, 5600 Fishers Lane, Rockville, MD 20857; phone 301-443-6470, fax 301-443-8683.

[3] Editors' note: Most AIDS grants referred to NIMH are coded AZ and the Office of AIDS Programs handles grant monitoring, but a few grants may be assigned to one of the three NIMH Divisions for this purpose. See "The Award Process" by Roberts, this volume, for a further discussion of this process.

[4] Editors' note: Although these reviewers usually cannot vote unless they hold an appointment in the NIH Reviewers Reserve, they can address issues relevant to the scientific merit of your application.

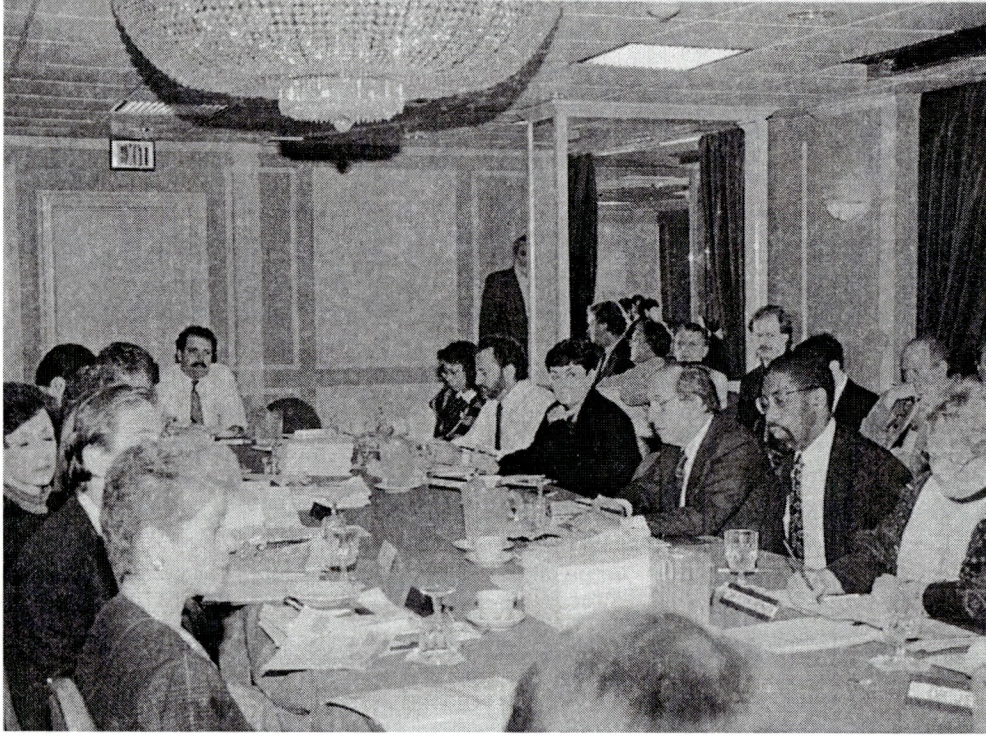

Figure 2. Members of the Mental Health Acquired Immunodeficiency Syndrome Research Review Committee (MHAZ) conducting a review meeting.

discussion of each application is full and fair, and the entire committee takes part in the review of each application.

Reviewing AIDS Applications

Different criteria may be applied during the review, depending on the type of grant application under consideration.[5] For regular research grants (R01s), these include significance, originality, adequacy of methodology, qualifications and experience of the principal investigator and staff, availability of resources, appropriateness of budget, and full and appropriate addressing of human subjects and animal issues. Each grant application generally has three reviewers who are specifically assigned to read and evaluate it. In addition, all IRG members are encouraged to read and comment on as many applications as possible outside their specific review assignments. At the review committee meeting, the assigned reviewers give their individual critiques, followed by an open discussion by the entire group. In unusual circumstances, should the committee determine that they need additional information or clarification of some point beyond that which was provided in the application, they can defer their decision and complete

[5] See "Selecting the Appropriate Research Mechanism" by Friedenberg *et al.*, this volume.

the review at the next meeting. The additional information may be obtained in writing in response to questions provided by the SRA, or a site visit may be required, although the latter is becoming less common in recent years.

At the end of that discussion, if the application contains "significant and substantial merit," reviewers individually assign scores for the application (described below).

Priority Scores and Percentiles

Priority scores are the most basic expression of the perceived quality of the application by the IRG. Applications are rated by each member of the standing IRG immediately following its discussion. As noted above, if an application is determined to have significant and substantial merit, it is given a score. Each member privately assigns a number from 1 to 5 (in 0.1 unit increments), 1 being the best and 5 the worst.

In order to provide scores that are as meaningful as possible and to provide stability and anchoring of the numerical values, descriptors have been developed with the assistance of a committee composed of psychometricians and other experts in evaluation processes. In developing the new descriptors, the group surveyed all the IRGs within the Institute. Table 1 is a reproduction of the poster that is used during the IRG meetings, and reviewers are advised to use these words to describe individual applications. In other words, if an application is truly outstanding (or excellent, or very good), the reviewers are asked to use that term and ultimately to vote a score that matches the word. Following the meeting, means are derived for each application, and the priority score is calculated by multiplying the mean by 100. This results in a score such as 132 or 277.

In order to encourage reviewers to continue to use the full range of scores, that is, to help prevent compression of scores toward the better end of the scale and to provide for better comparability between the various IRGs, a percentile is calculated for each application. The percentile becomes the principal, though not sole, basis for funding decisions. The calculation is done using the following formula, shown in (1): Percentiles are calculated on an IRG-by-IRG basis with the denominator (i.e., the "Number of Applications") being the total number of applications reviewed by that single committee during the current plus the previous two meetings. Priority scores for applications for the current review round are interdigitated with those from the two previous meetings of the IRG. The rank order of each appli-

Table 1. Priority Score Rating Scale	
Descriptor	Priority Score Range
Outstanding	1.0–1.5
Excellent	1.5–2.0
Very Good	2.0–2.5
Good	2.5–3.5
Acceptable	3.5–5.0

cation in that pool is then used in the formula. Applications rated NRFC are included in the denominator.

$$\text{Percentile} = \frac{\text{Rank Order} - 0.5}{\text{Number of Applications}} * 100 \tag{1}$$

Notification of Outcome of the Review

Within 5 days of the IRG meeting, a computer-generated letter is sent to each principal investigator informing him or her of the outcome of the review. The letter states the priority score and percentile for the application or NRFC, as the case may be.

Summary Statement[6]

Once the initial review is finished, the assigned reviewers revise their written comments to reflect any changes that resulted from discussion of the application, and written comments are also obtained from other (non-assigned) committee members who had substantive participation in the discussion. The revised critiques and other notes are given to the SRA, who uses them along with his or her notes taken during the meeting to prepare the summary statement. You should receive your summary statement within 7 or 8 weeks of the IRG meeting.

After reviewing your summary statement, if you think that there was a procedural mistake or a factual error that adversely affected the outcome of the review, you should communicate, either informally by a phone call to the program staff person assigned to your application or more formally by way of a letter to the program person with a copy to the SRA. Staff will consider your communication, probably sharing it with some of the reviewers and asking for their opinion. They may also discuss it with others within the Institute as necessary and appropriate. In those cases where it is determined that there was an error in the review, the application will be re-reviewed, either by the original IRG supplemented with additional reviewer expertise or by a different committee, as dictated by the situation. If an application is re-reviewed, it is important to remember that the same application is re-reviewed without modification.

In most cases, however, "disagreements" between the applicant and the IRG are scientific differences of opinion. In these situations, the committee's recommendation stands. In either case, we will discuss the sequence of events and the options with you. Ultimately, the burden of convincing the committee, that is, the IRG or study section, is on the applicant. Therefore, such differences of opinion are usually best dealt with in a revised application in which the investigator responds to the criticisms with additional data to support the validity of the proposed research, clarification of portions of the application that may have been misunderstood or inadequately presented, modifications to the application, or other approaches seen as appropriate by the applicant.

Council Review

At this point, the review process is still not complete. We have what is known as "dual review" because, in addition to the first level of review by the IRGs, there is a second level of review by National Advisory

---

[6] Editors' note: See "Reading between the Lines of Your Summary Statement" by Lyman, this volume.

Table 2. Dual Review System

First Level of Review
Initial Review Group or Study Section
    provides initial scientific review of grant applications
    does not set program priorities
    makes budget recommendations but no funding decisions

Second Level of Review
Council
    assesses quality of SRA review of grant applications
    makes recommendations on funding to Institute staff
    evaluates program priorities and relevance
    advises on policy

Mental Health Council (see Table 2).[7] This is a formally constituted and legally mandated body of scientists and lay people who have an interest in issues related to mental health and who have been appointed by the Secretary of the Department of Health and Human Services. Council meets three times a year to review the summary statements from the most recent round of IRG reviews and to determine, in essence, whether the review process was carried out properly. All concerns raised by applicants are brought to the attention of Council.

In most cases, Council concurs with IRG recommendations. However, if they observe that the review was flawed, they will recommend re-review. While they do not have the authority to change the priority score or the percentile on any application, they may draw attention of the Institute to an application that is of significant relevance to the Institute's programs.

Because Council action is required in order for the Institute to pay grants, it is not until Council has concurred with the IRG and staff recommendations or has made their own that the review process is considered complete.

Timeframe for the Review Process

For regular grants, the normal timeframe from receipt of the application to award is usually 9 to 10 months. Thus, applications received for the October/November receipt dates would go to IRG review in February and to Council in May, so that the earliest start date would be July 1. For AIDS applications there is an expedited process by which a receipt-to-award period does not exceed 6 months.[8] This has been mandated by Congress. So if you respond to a January 2 (AIDS) deadline, your application would be reviewed by the IRG in March and by Council in May, so that if your application received a favorable review, funding could begin in June. After Council review, you should talk to program staff members in order to learn about your funding status.[9]

---

[7] Editors' note: Fellowships and small grants are not reviewed by the Council.

[8] Editors' note: The expedited receipt dates for AIDS grants are January 2, May 1, and September 1, although you should check with NIMH staff members, as some mechanisms use different dates.

[9] For those proposing to do AIDS research, the program staff are members of the Office on AIDS.

Resubmission

If you believe you can write a better application, based on the review committee's critique, the best way to address your disagreement with aspects of the summary statement is to revise your application and resubmit it. Provide the best evidence, such as additional data, in support of your position, and do whatever you can to strengthen your application.

If you feel the summary statement is factually incorrect, you should study the summary statement carefully before you attempt to refute statements. Consider whether any of the comments have merit, but do not interpret criticisms as recommendations to make specific changes. Any changes you make in your application should be based on your best judgment as a scientist and researcher and not simply on a criticism by the IRG. Keep in mind that the criticisms in your summary statement represent the collective scientific opinion of the committee, not necessarily fact. (If we knew the answers, we would not need to do the research.) Nonetheless, the comments are from reputable scientists and deserve full and serious consideration.

Review Committee Participation

Now that you have an overview of the review process, you may be interested in serving on a review committee. This is an excellent way to serve your field as well as to learn about the review process firsthand. The NIH Consultant File has been developed and is maintained as a source of potential reviewers. In addition to information about potential reviewers' expertise and educational and professional background, data are maintained on publication record, ethnic background, age, and gender. With this tool, we are able to identify the required expertise as well as ensure that other factors are balanced as well. You can contact any staff member of NIMH (or NIH for that matter) if you wish to be listed in the Consultant File.

Summary

To summarize briefly the highlights of the process (which is usually completed within 9 months for regular applications and 6 months for AIDS grant applications), an application is received by DRG within NIH and assigned to an Institute and an IRG. The review committee evaluates the scientific and technical merit of the application and assigns it a priority score if, in their judgment, it contains significant and substantial merit. The priority score is translated into a percentile score. The application is reviewed by Council to ensure that the initial review process has been fairly and equitably carried out. Funding decisions are then made within the program divisions of the Institute, based largely on the percentile along with relevance to the program, mission of the Institute, and availability of funds.

Applicants are strongly encouraged to consult with DEA staff during the initial review phase, particularly if they are concerned with the assignment or other aspects of the review. Some individuals are mistakenly concerned that they may jeopardize the outcome of the review and the likelihood of funding of their application if they call too early or make remarks that might be viewed as critical. It is important that we dispel that misunderstanding. We are here to serve you. Do not hesitate to call or write us if you have any concern, and we will do out best to respond.

5

Selecting the Appropriate Research Mechanism

Eleanor Friedenberg, Thomas R. N. Lalley, Barry Lebowitz, and Steven Zalcman

The Public Health Service uses at least 130 mechanisms to support a variety of research activities. It is important to match the mechanism to both the investigator and the study. The section entitled "mechanisms" in the Program Announcement (PA) will tell you which mechanisms can be used in responding to it. We will focus here primarily on those mechanisms used by the NIMH AIDS research program.

Support Mechanisms

Mechanisms of support generally fall into three categories: (1) research training, (2) research scientist development, and (3) research grants. We will briefly discuss some highlights within each category, with particular focus on the predominant category—research grants.

Research Training

NIMH support for research training helps to enlarge the number of scientists conducting mental health research through grants to predoctoral and postdoctoral individuals (F31 and F32, respectively) and to institutions (T32). Some of the research training mechanisms, such as postdoctoral training grants, may be of particular interest to people who are relatively new in the field. Those with more experience may want broad information about NIMH research training opportunities to share with early career investigators that they are encouraging to pursue a research career.

Research training mechanisms range from the Minority Access to Research Careers (MARC) program, which literally can begin in high school and extend throughout the career, to individual and institutional pre- and postdoctoral research training grant awards. There is also the Minority Supplement Program that permits funds to supplement an existing research grant in order to develop the research career of a minority investigator.[1]

Research Scientist Development

The mechanisms called "research scientist development" (K awards) offer support at several levels for the development of researchers who have already completed the formal educational process. The support mechanisms range from Research Scientist Development Awards (for clinicians or researchers very early in their research careers) to Research Scientist Awards for more seasoned investigators. Support is offered to obtain research experience in a structured setting, with specific career goals outlined in the grant application and a specific mentor/mentee relationship for those who are not ready to conduct research independently.

NIMH also has three academic awards, which are specifically designed to further develop faculty members as lead researchers in their university settings. These awards are for psychiatrists and nurses only, in three specific program areas—children and adolescents, geriatrics, and schizophrenia—but they could be tied to AIDS work in those areas.

Research Grants

NIMH supports research through a variety of mechanisms focused on many basic and clinical research areas. There is a compilation of the current announcements of areas and programs for which NIMH now offers funding.[2] Although some Program Announcements are subject-specific, they indicate that support can be requested under several mechanisms, such as the R01 (the regular research grant), the R03 (the small grant), or the R29 (the FIRST award)—all of which are described below.

Regular Research Grant

The investigator-initiated research grant (R01) is the primary research support mechanism. The majority of NIMH research funding is committed to the R01 mechanism, which initially funds a research study for up to 5 years, although the grant can be extended through competitive renewal.

---

[1] Editors' note: This Program Announcement is described on pg 25 of "Program Announcements and Requests for Applications: Signals to the Field" by Pequegnat, this volume.

[2] Editors' note: See the listing in "Program Announcements and Requests for Applications: Signals to the Field" (Pequegnat, this volume).

Small Grant

The R03—the small-grant mechanism—is of particular interest to two groups of people: (1) relatively new researchers who are testing their ideas in conducting targeted research but for a shorter period of time; and (2) more experienced investigators who want to pilot an idea before requesting funds for a larger study.

The small-grant mechanism has two attractive features. First, it is reviewed on a more expedited review schedule than other research grants because it does not go to the second level of review, the National Advisory Mental Health Council. A person who applies for a small grant will be informed in a relatively short period of time whether it will be funded. A second attractive feature is that, recently, the financial and temporal limits on small grants were liberalized. A small grant now may be requested for up to $50,000 in direct costs yearly for up to 2 years (previously it was a $25,000 award for 1 year).

First Investigator Research Support Transition (FIRST)

The FIRST (First Investigator Research Support Transition) grant (R29) is an award mechanism limited to less-experienced investigators (those not more than 5 years past the doctorate degree) who may not have had an R01 or are trying to make the transition from being a co-investigator to a principal investigator. FIRST applicants may have had an R03 but not an R01. Applications may be requested for 5 years only. It is nonrenewable and has a $350,000 cap on direct costs over the 5-year award period, but it is a perfect mechanism for people who are not ready to compete with more fully experienced researchers for the regular R01 grants.[3]

Program Projects and Center Grants

There is another series of mechanisms in the research category, which we will only briefly mention: program projects (P01) and center grants (P50). These mechanisms are for more experienced investigators who have mobilized a large multidisciplinary team. If you are an early career investigator, it would be to your advantage to contact some of the research centers supported by NIMH. It may be possible to negotiate individual support under the sponsorship of a center related to a specific area.[4]

Cooperative Agreements

The cooperative agreement (U01) is a mechanism in which NIMH staff and researchers in the field collaborate, with NIMH staff functioning as co-investigators. Cooperative agreements are issued as RFAs and request that the applicant follow specific directives for applying. NIMH is currently supporting a cooperative agreement, an AIDS multisite clinical trial to test preventive interventions with multiple populations.

---

[3] Editors' note: At the review committee the R29s are reviewed in a block, often before the R01s, and different review criteria apply.

[4] Editors' note: In fiscal year 1995, NIMH was providing support to five AIDS Research Centers.

Advice on Research Mechanisms

The NIMH staff can be helpful in clarifying how these and other mechanisms can be used to meet your needs. In addition, the staff in the AIDS program can give you guidance about how these mechanisms are used to develop knowledge in the field of HIV infection and AIDS.

Review Criteria

For each support mechanism there are specific evaluation criteria. Thus, the NIMH AIDS review committee, which reviews applications across all support mechanisms, groups by mechanism the applications during review to ensure that the appropriate criteria are applied. As you prepare a research grant or develop an application, examine the section called "Review Criteria" in the PA, because the committee will apply those criteria as they review your application.

What Your Grant Application Number Means

What follows in this section is a breakdown of a sample grant application number, 1 R01 MH10000-04 S1A1.

					Suffixes		
Application type	**Activity code**	**Administrative organization**	**Serial number**	*Grant year*[5]	*Supplement*	*Amendment*	*Allowance*
1	R01	MH	10000	-04	S1	A1	n/a

Application Type

A single-digit code identifying the type of application received and processed.

1   New
2   Competing Continuation
3   Supplement
4   Extension
5   Noncompeting Continuation
6   Change of Institute or Division (new, training programs)
7   Change of Grantee or Training Institution
8   Change of Institute or Division (noncompeting continuation)
9   Change of Institute or Division (competing continuation)

---

[5] An additional four-digit suffix may appear in a grant identification number recorded in the CRISP System, to identify separate projects.

Activity Code

A three-digit code identifies a specific mechanism of extramural activity. The major categories are:

F   Fellowship
K   Research Career Programs
R   Research Projects
P   Program Projects and Center
T   Training Projects

The description of the specific mechanisms appears on pages 60–63.

Administrative Organization

A two-letter code identifying the first major-level subdivision. In the example above, "MH" refers to the National Institute of Mental Health (NIMH). The codes for other Institutes appear on page 60.

Serial Number

A five-digit number generally assigned sequentially within an Institute or Division.

Suffixes

Grant Year A two-digit number indicating the actual segment or budget period of a project. The grant year number (01, 02, etc.) is preceded by a dash, to separate it from the serial number (e.g., MH 00900-04). The grant year number is incremented by one for each succeeding renewal. Thus, the -04 year suffix above indicates that this is the fourth grant year.

Supplement The letter "S" and related number identifying a particular supplemental record (e.g., S1, S2). Supplement designations follow the grant year or the amendment designation, as the case may be (e.g., MH 00900-04A1S1).

Amendment The letter "A" and related number identifying each amended application (e.g., A1, A2, etc.). Amendment designations follow the grant year or the supplement designation, as the case may be (e.g., MH 34567-02A1).

Allowance The letter "X" and related number identifies a fellowship's institutional allowance record. Allowance designations also follow the grant year or other designation.

Codes Used for the Institutes

AA   National Institute on Alcohol Abuse and Alcoholism (NIAAA)
AG   National Institute on Aging (NIA)
AL   National Institute of Allergy and Infectious Diseases (NIAID)
AR   National Institute of Arthritis and Musculoskeletal and Skin Diseases (NIAMS)

CA	National Cancer Institute
CL	Clinical Center (CLC)
CT	Division of Computer Research and Technology (DCRT)
DA	National Institute on Drug Abuse (NIDA)
DC	National Institute on Deafness and other Communication Disorders (NIDCD)
DE	National Institute of Dental Research (NIDR)
DK	National Institute of Diabetes and Digestive and Kidney Diseases (NIDDK)
DS	Division of Safety (DS-ORS-OD)
ES	National Institute of Environmental Health Sciences (NIEHS)
EY	National Eye Institute (NIE)
GM	National Institute of General Medical Sciences (NIGMS)
HD	National Institute of Child Health and Human Development (NICHD)
HG	National Center for Human Genome Research (NCHGR)
HL	National Heart, Lung, and Blood Institute (NHLBI)
LM	National Library of Medicine (NLM)
MH	National Institute of Mental Health (NIMH)
NR	National Institute for Nursing Research (NINR)
NS	National Institute for Neurological Disorders and Stroke (NINDS)
OD	Office of the Director (NIH)
RG	Division of Research Grants (DRG)
RR	National Center for Research Resources (NCRR)
TW	Fogarty International Center (FIC)

Fellowship Programs

F 30—Individual Predoctoral NRSA for M.D./Ph.D. Fellowships Individual fellowships for predoctoral training that leads to the combined M.D./Ph.D. degrees.

F 31—Predoctoral Individual National Research Service Award Provides predoctoral individuals with supervised research training in specified health and health-related areas leading toward the research degree (e.g., Ph.D.)

F 32—Postdoctoral Individual National Research Service Award Provides postdoctoral research training to individuals in order to broaden their scientific background and extend their potential for research in specified health-related areas.

F 34—MARC NRSA Faculty Fellowships Available to selected faculty members from minority institutions in order to enable them to obtain advanced training in specified health and health-related areas.

Research Career Programs

K 02—Research Scientist Development Award–Research For support of a scientist, committed to research, in need of additional experience.

K 05—Research Scientist Award For the support of a research scientist qualified to pursue independent research that would extend the research program of the sponsoring institution or to direct an essential part of this research program.

K 07—Academic/Teacher Award To create and encourage a stimulating approach to disease curricula that will attract high-quality students, foster academic career development of promising young teacher-investigators, develop and implement excellent multidisciplinary curricula through interchange of ideas, and enable the grantee institution to strengthen its existing teaching program. Only supported in areas of aging, children, and schizophrenia in NIMH.

K 20—Scientist Development Award for Clinicians To foster the development of outstanding scientists with potential to make important contributions to the fields of alcoholism, drug abuse, or mental health research. Primarily intended to provide supervised research experience for clinically trained individuals, especially physicians, who show special promise for a research career but do not possess sufficient research skills.

K 21—Scientist Development Award To foster development of outstanding scientists with potential for making important contributions to the fields of alcoholism, drug abuse, or mental health research. Primarily intended to meet the need for supervised research experience for highly promising biological or behavioral scientists who need further supervised research experience.

Research Projects

R 01—Research Project (Traditional) To support a discrete, specified, circumscribed project to be performed by the named investigator(s) in an area representing his or her specific interest and competencies.

R 03—Small Research Grants To provide research support specifically limited in time and amount for studies in categorical program areas. Small grants provide flexibility for initiating studies that are generally for preliminary short-term projects; they are nonrenewable.

R 10—Cooperative Clinical Research (Grants) To support clinical evaluation of various methods of therapy and/or prevention in specific disease areas. These represent cooperative programs between participating institutions and principal investigators and are usually conducted under established protocols.

R 13—Conferences (Traditional) To support international or national meetings, conferences, and workshops.

R 29—First Independent Research Support and Transition (FIRST) Award To provide a sufficient initial period of research support for newly independent biomedical investigators to develop their research capabilities and demonstrate the merit of their research ideas.

R 37—Method to Extend Research in Time (MERIT) Award To provide long-term support to investigators whose research competence and productivity are distinctly superior and who are highly likely to continue to perform in an outstanding manner. Investigators may not apply for a MERIT award. Program staff and/or members of the cognizant National Advisory Council/Board will identify candidates for the MERIT award during the course of reviewing competing research grants applications prepared and submitted in accordance with regular PHS requirements.

R 43—Small Business Innovation Research Grants (SBIR)-Phase I To support projects limited in time and amount to establish the technical merit and feasibility of R&D ideas that may ultimately lead to a commercial product(s) or service(s).

R 44—Small Business Innovation Research Grants (SBIR)-Phase II To support in-depth development of R&D ideas whose feasibility has been established in Phase I and which are likely to result in commercial products or services.

R 55—James A. Shannon Director's Award To provide a limited award to investigators to further develop, test, and refine research techniques; perform secondary analysis of available data sets; test the feasibility of innovative and creative approaches; and conduct other discrete projects that can demonstrate their research capabilities and lend additional weight to their already meritorious applications.

Training Programs

T 32—Institutional National Research Service Award To enable institutions to establish and conduct research training programs and make National Research Service Awards to individuals selected by them for predoctoral and/or postdoctoral research training in specified shortage areas.

T 34—MARC Undergraduate NRSA Institutional Grants To enable minority institutions to make National Research Service Awards to individuals selected by them for undergraduate research training in the biomedical and behavioral sciences.

T 35—NRSA Short-Term Research Training To provide individuals with research training during off-quarters or summer periods to encourage research careers and/or research in areas of national need.

Cooperative Agreements

U 01—Research Project (Cooperative Agreements) To support a discrete, specified, circumscribed project to be performed by the named investigator(s) in an area representing their specific interest and competencies. Institute staff are co-investigators.

U 10—Cooperative Clinical Research (Cooperative Agreements) To support clinical evaluation of various methods of therapy and/or prevention in specific disease areas. These represent cooperative programs between participating institutions and principal investigators and are usually conducted under established protocols.

General Grantsmanship Guidelines

Now that you are familiar with the kinds of research mechanisms available for conducting AIDS research, we would like to share some tips on how to obtain that funding.

Do Not Play the Odds

First, in selecting support mechanisms, do not attempt to play the odds. Beginning investigators are sometimes advised that they should apply for R01 grants rather than R03 small grants because they might compete with more experienced individuals for small grants and because there may be less funding available for small grants than for R01s.

That advice is misleading. A mechanism of support should be selected based on your career research goals. You are well advised to use the one that is most appropriate for what you want to do, how long your project will take, and where you are in your professional development. Playing the odds of an R01 versus an R03 is a no-win game because the probabilities of funding change from year to year in ways that cannot be anticipated. You should be concerned about which mechanism is most appropriate for you and your proposed project.

Consult with NIMH Program Staff

Consult extensively with NIMH program staff before you submit your grant application. Instead of trying to figure out the NIMH system by discussing strategies with your colleagues, consult with NIMH about the best approach for you, based on their knowledge of the system. Most of us at NIMH like nothing better than to be asked intelligent questions that permit us to be helpful to people.

By seeking staff counsel before you apply for a grant, you will avoid having your application become an "orphan grant"—one that is submitted without any prior contact with program staff. We still receive applications from investigators who could have saved years of effort if they had simply called and taken advantage of the knowledge and expertise of our staff.

It may be useful to obtain NIMH consultation on the budget. If you justify everything in your proposed budget, there is a chance that the review committee may cut items, but if you have not justified everything, the IRG will certainly recommend a cut.

Think Small; Think FIRST

If you are an inexperienced investigator you should "think small"; start with a small grant and do a pilot study. NIMH receives proposals from new investigators requesting $4 million a year, and from people who have 5 years of good clinical work and no research experience asking for $3 million over 5 years. These proposals are unlikely to be recommended for funding.

The small grant is designed primarily for investigators who: (1) do not have enough preliminary data to submit a proposal for a competitive regular research grant, (2) do not have extensive research experience to demonstrate the ability to provide scientific leadership for a large research project, or (3) are located in institutions without well-developed research traditions or resources. Success in generating interesting, useful data from the small grant would clearly enhance the likelihood of obtaining funding for a subsequent FIRST or an R01.

Play from Strength

Submit a research application in an area in which you are well-trained and have a good idea. Many potential applicants believe that in order to conduct NIMH-funded research your proposal must fit within an existing NIMH Program Announcement (PA) or Request for Application (RFA). That assumption is incorrect. NIMH issues many PAs indicating its interest in supporting specific research programs and program areas. They are issued for many reasons as mechanisms to stimulate awareness in the fields, not as a constraint for NIMH research awards. The Institute remains strongly committed to supporting excellent investigator-initiated research, as long as the proposed study is consistent with the overall NIMH mental health research mission.

Provide Pilot Data

You must have pilot data in your application to demonstrate that your study is feasible. To fund the pilot study, obtain an NIMH small grant first, tap your university's small grants fund, or seek out the sponsorship of a research center, of which there are many kinds.

Expose Your Logic

In the process of developing a research project, you make many decisions. Do not write a proposal as if it were a journal article where you are succinctly reporting your results. Rather, show reviewers that you considered several options, rejected one, and chose the other. For example, indicate your awareness of the available research instruments by providing a rationale for the instrument that you selected and stating why you rejected the others as inappropriate.

Explore Research Scientist Development Support

Many prospective applicants have heavy teaching or clinical responsibilities. If you face this pressure, consider applying for career development support. Career development awards allow you to concentrate on developing your research career and be freed up from clinical or teaching responsibilities. We have mechanisms that can permit you to have a full-time research career for the rest of your life.

Persevere

If you are not successful in obtaining support after the first submission of your research application, be prepared to revise and resubmit. Forty percent of the grants funded in fiscal year 1990 had been submitted more than one time. If you resubmit, your success rate is likely to be improved because you have responded to the previous review committee's critique provided in the summary statement.

Fundamental Review Questions

In the review of any project grant, whether it is a FIRST award, an R03, or an R01, the committee asks three fundamental questions:

- ✔ How good are the ideas you are seeking to test?
- ✔ How well-designed are the experiments you have proposed to conduct in order to test those ideas?

✔ How capable are you to serve as the principal investigator in carrying out the proposed experiments?

The step-by-step process outlined in this handbook should permit you to demonstrate to the NIMH reviewers that you have good ideas and that you are capable of testing in experiments that will contribute to knowledge in AIDS research.

6

Selecting Issues and Hypotheses for a Research Proposal

Spero M. Manson

Whenever you write a grant proposal, several questions usually cross your mind: Have I chosen the right topic? Is this a fundable issue? Is this important research? Those questions come up frequently, and they have served as the genesis for the following commentary on the process of identifying and capitalizing on the recognition of a critical research issue.

There is a natural history, a cycle if you will, of ideas and issues that is important to keep in mind when trying to answer these questions. There are seven major forces that I feel shape this cycle, which are the focus of this chapter.

An important part of the process of identifying a critical issue is to conduct an ethnographic study of the funding culture. In that regard, I am going to discuss my perception of NIMH as a culture and of charitable and private foundations as cultures. Then, I will review the tools that you should use to identify these critical issues, as well as some of the mechanisms by which you can maintain this effort on an ongoing basis. This is a constant effort, but it can be interesting, even exciting.

Catching the Wave

Ideas and issues, I believe, have a point of initial introduction, reach a threshold of recognition, and then wane. The degree of interest in a particular issue may be due to the field of study, or it may be a function of the agenda of a funding agency. We will talk about it in both senses.

If you were to plot this wave of interest in an issue, you would find that there is a specific time frame during which you can access this interest. You can mark this time in months, fiscal quarters, fiscal years, even in terms of careers, but the wave is actually continuous. There comes a point, the threshold of recognition, when a critical mass of resources and energy builds behind an issue and captures the popular imagination. The amplitude of the wave may be different from one type of issue to another, but it remains ascended for a period of time, then gradually loses force over time. The same issue may reappear a decade or two later.

The challenge in selecting a critical issue is figuring out how to catch a wave on its ascent. I think a surfing analogy is appropriate. If you try to catch a wave too early, it will not carry you to shore but will go right past you. On the other hand, if you catch the wave too late, it may crash on top of you. Therefore, you want to catch the wave not at its exact peak, but at its greatest momentum. The key, then, is to determine the size of the wave, how quickly it will be moving through time, and when it might end.

There have been a number of waves during my career. With respect to AIDS and mental health–related disorders, we are at the point of greatest momentum. Therefore, your timing with respect to this particular set of issues is good, and thus, potentially fruitful.

Ten years ago, even five years ago, the wave was just beginning to build. At that time, you could have formulated the best ideas in terms of AIDS and its mental health implications, but because it was early in the developmental history of that wave, your ideas would not have experienced the same reception.

However, during the next three to five years, much of the major work in AIDS research already may well be under way. Many of the major efforts will have already caught the wave; it may even begin declining with respect to some of these areas. It is important for you to think about this, not just in terms of your work related to HIV infection and mental health disorders, but as it applies to other interests.

You also should remember that these waves may move through different institutes at different times. Therefore, if you drew the wave of interest in HIV research in various fields, you might not see them as overlapping.

The question, then, is how do I describe and how do I catch a wave? This can be answered by reviewing the seven forces that can make things happen for you at the peak of that wave: (1) need, (2) feasibility, (3) generalizability (not in the scientific sense, but in a programmatic sense), (4) continuity, (5) applicability, (6) scientific merit, and (7) fundability.

Need

The questions that pertain to need are: To whom is this issue important? Who has a stake in it? What is the nature of their stake in the field? What do they perceive as the benefits from the systematic investigation of this particular issue?

Need is mercurial, because it changes depending on the person to whom you are talking. The degree of perceived need is not the same for one constituency as it is for another. The definition of need for the person in the street, who may be infected with HIV or know someone who is, may be quite different than that of a politician, scientist, or staff person at a funding agency. It is important to recognize that the definition or perception of need varies depending upon the person and the setting.

In my experience, one of the most common mistakes that many of us make when we work in this field is in thinking that granting agencies perceive need in the same way as those with whom we work. We act based on our assumptions of need, and we do not take the time and effort to check the concordance of perceptions of need.

When people visiting my program say, "We need to research this problem because we need answers to these questions," I ask, "Well, who else do you think needs this? Are there other people like yourselves, as well as other agencies or organizations, that perceive this need as equally important as you do? In what way do they perceive it as a need?" Answers to each of these questions help us to describe a wave.

Feasibility

Another consideration in catching the wave at its optimal point has to do with feasibility. There may be consensus that an issue is critical, but we must assess feasibility: Are there available methods to pursue this critical issue in some systematic fashion that will answer the questions that underpin the need? It may be, for example, that while need is high, we may lack the methods, the design, the instrumentation, or the analytic techniques to be able productively to ask questions that will address that need. When those things are not synchronous, the wave begins to oscillate and we cannot catch it.

Feasibility has to do not only with the status of the field, but also with your personal readiness. You must consider whether it is feasible for you, at given points in your career, to invest the time and energy to pursue the study of this critical issue to its logical outcome. You must make a personal assessment about whether HIV infection and mental health–related issues are relevant to you and how you project your career. Because of other demands, such as teaching, clinical responsibilities, or new administrative assignments, it may not be timely for you to pursue a given opportunity.

On the other hand, such an analysis may confirm that this is the appropriate time for you to pursue this need. Thus, feasibility must be assessed both from the viewpoint of the field and your personal situation in order to catch that wave. Then, you must assess how to obtain the necessary resources.

Generalizability

Another force in catching this wave is related to generalizability: How does this issue link with other issues? Is this an isolated issue that is independent of others?

If the answer to this second question is "yes," then your issue is relatively insulated from other kinds of issues. In that case, it is likely to be short-lived and fail to carry you into related areas.

Also, generalizability has to do with the programmatic salience or need of the issue. Is this issue going to be meaningful not only to other investigators but also to other people who have administrative and programmatic responsibility? To the extent that the interest in this issue generalizes into other areas of responsibility, the longer that wave is likely to last and to advance.

Continuity

Continuity is a permutation of generalizability, but it relates to your career path. Last year at NIMH, there were between 30 and 50 new funding initiatives. Each one of those new initiatives represents a wave; there were 30, 40, or 50 waves suddenly rippling through NIMH and its programmatic funding. Which one will you attempt to catch in terms of linking your work and interests to it?

One needs to be very thoughtful about this analysis because the wave you want to catch is the one that will carry you forward into the next wave, linking you to others, and ensuring some continuity to your career and program of research. One of the dangers of multiple opportunities is not conducting a careful analysis that will permit you to develop a program of research addressing a set of critical issues that spans funding opportunities. Otherwise, you may find yourself always studying a new set of issues in a new field that consumes an enormous amount of energy.

Applicability

The most difficult force to capture and sustain is one that does not have an apparent applicability, at least in the immediate future. For the most part, the populations within which we work want to see the results applied in a way that help people. While they permit some grace period, continued access and the ability to work with populations of interest to us determine whether or not we can catch that wave and how far we can take it.

Scientific Merit

The majority of investigators seem to believe that they must employ only the most sophisticated survey or experimental methods in order to be judged adequate in terms of scientific merit. There are many instances where qualitative research techniques are important and may be the only way to address questions effectively.[1] Some of you may feel that qualitative research techniques are not rigorous enough to survive review. These concerns may be valid, because peer review committees, for example, seldom have investigators who are expert in qualitative research techniques. They are more likely to be expert in other types of quantitatively oriented methods.

 The challenge, then, is to develop a design that will either blend the strengths of both or to make the case that, in fact, qualitative techniques can be reviewed using the same criteria and standards as the quantitative techniques. This can be done. You must address the issue of scientific merit and illustrate how you can use the available techniques to study the critical issues posed in your research. Otherwise, you may find yourself at either end of the wave rather than catching its momentum.

Fundability

The seventh major force, which I deliberately have placed last, has to do with fundability. In my experience, fundability is often at the top of the list of considerations in developing a proposal. It usually is the first question asked: "Can I get this funded?"

However, if fundability serves as the primary motive in selecting a critical issue to study, there is the risk that your career will have no continuity. You run the risk of studying a variety of interesting research questions, but may not contribute to a program of research.

Some of the best work I have performed has been with little or no money. This may be because I was forced to be parsimonious and innovative in my thinking. I had the opportunity to stretch the bounds of what I was trying to do. Then, the challenge became figuring out how I could continue to pursue this line of study in a way that was fundable. So, fundability does indeed play an important role, but hopefully, does not serve as a *raison d'etre* for selecting a particular issue.

Drawing the Wave

There are systematic ways by which you can gather the information to assess the forces creating the wave you would like to catch. Consider becoming an anthropologist and conducting an ethnography of the funding agencies that provide support. There is a culture at NIMH different from the cultures at NIAAA and NIDA; it is important to be aware of those differences. They each have a different set of beliefs and sense of priority and mission, despite clear areas of overlap.

How can you discover these cultures, and thereby increase the likelihood of success in pursuing your research? There is no way in which, despite your best efforts, you can keep abreast of all the changes and fluctuations within NIMH, NIDA, or NIAAA. You, therefore, need to develop a Dr. Parron, a Dr. Stover, or a Dr. Pequegnat as your advocate within the Institute. They can explain the basic beliefs, logic, and language of the Institute. They also can provide information, though available to everybody, but which most researchers wait to receive rather than solicit directly from program officers.

[1] See "Qualitative Inquiry: An Underutilized Strategy in AIDS Research" by Pequegnat *et al.,* this volume.

You are equally important to your advocacy because project officers are like investment brokers. They make an investment in you. They gamble that they can bring you through the phase of proposal development and, hopefully, to the next phase: a funded proposal. To the extent that this happens, they will have succeeded not only in personal terms, but also programmatically and they will be rewarded.

Another important way to gather information is to volunteer for professional activities. One example is to volunteer to review for conferences or journal articles. This allows you to preview work likely to surface in a year or two. It is a wonderful educational opportunity and offers a better sense of where the wave is and how you might access it.

Useful Tools

There are a number of tools that can help you to identify critical issues and assess where your interests lie with respect to a potential wave.

Current Contents

One tool is *Current Contents,* a weekly publication that prints the tables of contents of the major journals in a variety of fields. For example, the Social and Behavioral Science edition of *Current Contents* publishes the tables of contents for over a thousand journals. In 15 minutes a week I am able to identify, by title, the major articles relevant to my work and to assess which issues to pursue. Your university and many public libraries subscribe to *Current Contents.* The subscription cost is only $190 a year and it is worth a personal subscription if the publication is not available through institutional resources. It is even tax deductible.

Review Articles

Contemporary Psychology, Contemporary Sociology, and annual reviews of the social and behavioral sciences are great sources to pursue. Major debates and lines of inquiring are synthesized, representing an efficient way to update your knowledge. Most major libraries subscribe to these sources; you should review them on a regular basis. An example specific to this substantive area is International AIDS Conference abstracts.

Policy Documents

Policy documents are a third tool of enormous potential benefit. You probably have been told about some of the policy documents, both congressional and Institute-related, that have been issued in recent years with respect to AIDS. You should know that the Institute of Medicine and the U.S. Congressional Office of Technology Assessment both produce major policy documents. Review these for long-term trends that may result in program initiatives.

For example, publication of *Health and Behavior: New Frontiers for the Biobehavioral Sciences* by the Institute of Medicine in 1982 contributed to a series of NIMH programmatic initiatives. It is responsible for the founding of the Health and Behavior Branch and provided an impetus for prevention research. Reading this report, you could have anticipated some of the major programmatic emphases of the NIMH in the late 1980s.

In the AIDS arena there are several critical reports that can provide similar guidance. For example, the President's Commission on AIDS Research published an annual report. The National Academy of Sciences published several volumes, the last of which was *The Second Decade.*

There also are some other reports deserving review. The first is the *Annual Summary of PHS Grant Funding*, which compiles brief abstracts of all funded grants catalogued by Institutes, states, and often topics. The results of these efforts will not be published in the literature for another two to five years; these abstracts inform you of work in progress.

Newsletters

Another major source of current information is newsletters from major professional organizations and research groups. Programs such as the Directors of Mental State Health and Substance Abuse publish various newsletters. In the aggregate these newsletters can provide you with current and relevant information about issues from different perspectives.

Federal Publications

The contracts and summary report provides a review of all activities supported by this mechanism. Contracts are used for some projects because of the tight fiscal and administrative review controls. However, contracts may prove to be an advantage because of the less protracted review process and the opportunity to address specific questions of interest to both the investigator and sponsor.

Another reasonably up-to-date source are monograph series produced by each of the major Institutes. These monographs may be produced, released, and distributed more quickly than a typical book. Authors are likely to be the funded investigators from that Institute, providing additional insight into the investments by these Institutes.

Finally, the NIH *Public Advisory Group Book* is a critical tool. This document provides you with the name, institutional affiliation, and length of tenure of all of the members of the review groups. These persons are the peers who will judge your research applications. Determine their views on the critical research issues of the day by closely examining their publications.

Putting It Together

There are a variety of ways for implementing all of this. Develop an internal advocate to visit when in the vicinity of NIMH. Another resource can be found among your own institution resources. Every university has an office devoted to research services. They often see as many as 200 to 300 grants in a cycle, and therefore have a wealth of experience that remains untapped. Turn them into allies who can provide you with useful information pertinent to the development of your application.

The steps outlined in this handbook will, then, enable you to devise a research application that will allow you to catch the wave that will carry you through a productive and rewarding career as a research scientist.

7

Reading between the Lines of Your Summary Statement

William Lyman

The summary statement, which is sent to each prospective principal investigator, indicates how the proposal fared in the review process. Read by an informed investigator, it is not only a description of a past event but also a clue to the future—such as whether your proposal, as written, is likely to be funded or whether a revised and resubmitted application may succeed. I am going to describe what is in the summary statement (sometimes called the "pink sheet," because it formerly was printed on pink paper), how to interpret what it means about the probable fate of your proposal, and how you can influence (to some extent) your success rate as a grant applicant.

Enhancing Your Chances by Using the System

To increase your chances of a favorable and fundable outcome to the review process, it is important to be well-informed about the system and about those who will be assessing your proposal. One way is to determine which IRG is likely to be reviewing your proposal—even before you write it. If you are responding to an RFA (Request for an Application) or an RFP (Request for a Proposal), there might be some hint in terms of which Institute is sponsoring that solicitation. Certain Institutes will have only one or two IRGs that will review such applications. By checking the roster of reviewers on those IRGs, you can run a computer search of the members' publications and include in the literature review his or her work in your area.

As part of your advance intelligence, you can also obtain pink sheets (or modified pink sheets with certain personal information and priority scores deleted) from the IRG's former reviews by submitting a formal Freedom of Information (FOI) request to the Institute's FOI officer.[1] Those pink sheets will give

---

[1] Editors' note: While it is possible to obtain sanitized funded grant applications and summary statements, this is a lengthy process. It may be more efficient to solicit experience from colleagues and NIMH staff.

you some indication of how that IRG has reviewed a given set of proposals. You can also obtain the proposals through the Institute's FOI officer. This information may help you improve or enrich your grant application by giving you a different perspective about what is expected of you. Another excellent way is to volunteer to become a reviewer, which will expose you to many research applications and to the review process.

Interpreting the Pink Sheet

When you receive your pink sheet, you will find that there is considerable information to be gleaned from it—especially between the lines. Of course, if you discover that your proposal was approved unanimously, received a priority score of 100, and is in the first percentile, you will never need to read between the lines; you will simply read the bottom line.[2] If the budget you proposed is unchanged, there is little need to pore over the pink sheet. Simply celebrate!

But if the outcome was less than ideal, you may need to read the summary statement much more closely. The "recommendation" section has been partially discussed already in terms of approval, and whether or not it is unanimous. There is a tendency now to make votes unanimous whenever possible, because no reviewer wants to prepare a minority report unless a major scientific issue is at stake. If you have received unanimous approval, but a priority score in the 300s, for example, the complete pink sheet requires careful examination.

The "critique" is perhaps the most important portion of the summary statement in terms of what it may imply. You need to look at what has been written about what you have proposed and what has been deleted. For the most part the proposal's strengths will be emphasized in this section. Sometimes these remarks will seem somewhat gratuitous and patronizing. If you detect that tone ("damning with faint praise") in your pink sheet critique, it is cause for concern; other sections may reveal the reason.

If in discussing your experimental design, the summary contains phrases such as "overly ambitious," that, too, is cause for concern. Reviewers use that term to imply that the applicant's track record, amount of proposed effort, and institutional resources may indicate the proposed principal investigator is incapable of doing what has been proposed. The use of the words "overly ambitious" is telling you, in effect, that when you revise your grant application (as you will probably need to do), you should take a critical look at each section and scale it down.

For example, consider again the number and scope of the specific aims. There is a tendency to put too much in this section because you want to have your proposal appear to be comprehensive. As you reexamine your specific aims, make sure that each is focused and that each aim is not really two or three aims.

A key consideration is whether you have a hypothesis that can be tested. Proposals are severely damaged by not proposing a hypothesis. The first sentence of the grant application should begin, "The hypothesis I am going to test is . . . " It focuses your research application, and it focuses the reviewer.[3]

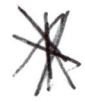Another important consideration should be the number of years of funding you are requesting. You may have initially submitted a proposal for 5 years of funding, but if your proposal was unfunded and you revise it and resubmit, consider a study for a shorter period of time. You can acknowledge that it is difficult to justify 5 years of work and ask to modify the project's duration to make it less ambitious and more feasible.

---

[2] Editors' note: For an explanation of a priority score and percentile, see "The Review Process" by Stamper, this volume.

[3] Editors' note: See "How Do You Formulate a Testable Exciting Hypothesis?" by Dawes, this volume.

If your proposal receives the terse recommendation of Not Recommended for Further Consideration (NRFC), it is very significant. This message is that your proposal has a fatal scientific flaw, either in its conceptualization from the hypothesis to be tested or in its methodology; there is something grossly in error. You cannot simply revise a small part of the proposal and hope it will go through; in fact, you should probably not resubmit.

Implications of the Priority Score

When the committee recommends approval of a proposal, it also expresses a level of enthusiasm—outstanding, excellent, and so forth—which is translated into a priority score (and ultimately into a percentile). If your proposal receives a priority score of 100 to 150 and an equally low percentile, it will almost certainly be funded.

A priority score between 220 and 240 will probably not receive a percentile that will permit funding, but the IRG is telling you that it is a good proposal, and you should be encouraged to resubmit a revised application, following closely the recommendations provided in the critique. If the committee receives a revised version of that application and they verify that you followed the recommended changes, the revised application may receive an approval with an improved score.[4]

If your proposal receives a score in the 300–350 range, the committee is telling you that it is potentially interesting, but needs a considerable amount of work. It may not be ready for the next submission deadline, but do not give up on it. Most people who get a score between 300 and 350 feel quite devastated. In truth, there is still reason to revise and resubmit.

If you receive a score between 400 and 450, even if you have a very competent and compassionate Scientific Review Administrator (SRA) who is focusing on positive aspects of your proposal, do not be misled into thinking that, with minor modifications, you can transform it into a fundable proposal. With scores in this range, the committee has not given a Not Recommended for Further Consideration (NRFC) because there was not a fatal flaw; however, they are suggesting that this proposal has severe methodological problems and it probably should not be resubmitted, unless you can really change it significantly.

Many applicants view a 450 score as an invitation to work very hard at a revision and resubmit. But more realistically, the proposal is probably so weak that your best effort can only improve it to about a 350 priority score. If the reviewers receive it a second time and it still scores in the 300s, it could have a negative effect on them, setting a tone that might not be in your best interest the next time you submit.

Rebuttal and Resubmission

You may or may not agree with the review committee's specific criticisms of your proposal. For example, many people proposing to do AIDS research will write that they plan to be doing *in vitro* immunologic tests. If the review group responds that these tests are not appropriate or they will not demonstrate *in vivo* possibilities as stated by the applicant, serious consideration should be given to that response. Some people may want to refute it when they resubmit their application. But if the criticism appears to be well-founded and has been discussed in an open forum, you may decide that you do not want to fight that point on the resubmission even if you feel the review may be incorrect.

---

[4] Editors' note: The "catch-22" is that your proposal may not be reviewed by the same set of reviewers. The new reviewers may identify problems with your research application that were not raised during the previous review.

In reviewing revisions, the IRG members have access to previous pink sheets (and do look at them), because they want to know whether and how the applicant has addressed the points raised by the earlier IRG. In the real world, reviewers may not have time to review your research application until the last minute, and it may not be reviewed under ideal circumstances in location or time. At such times, reviewers may place too much reliance upon the previous pink sheets. If that occurs, you may be able to detect it when you receive the latest pink sheet, and you have a right to appeal. If you believe you have addressed the initial issues but the summary statement argues that you have not, exercise your right to appeal.

In summary, my experience as a permanent member of a review committee has convinced me that the system symbolized by the pink sheet—peer review—works very well. Good proposals receive excellent reviews and therefore are later funded. Applicants who submit weak proposals are encouraged to resubmit and correct the flaws. If they do, their proposals are funded, too.

8

The Award Process

Sherry Roberts

As soon as potential grantees learn that the Initial Review Group (IRG) has met, the Office on AIDS begins to receive a flurry of phone calls and questions. In this chapter I have tried to address most of the typical questions as well as provide additional information that you may find useful.

When Are Funding Decisions Made?

Funding decisions are made three times a year after the meeting of the NIMH National Advisory Mental Health Council. If you have received a low percentile and Council approves your grant, you will then be considered for funding.

How Are Funding Decisions Made?

In each Program Announcement (PA) or Request for Application (RFA) there is a section called "Award Criteria," which is what the funding institute will use in making funding decisions. In most AIDS Program Announcements there are three basic award criteria: (1) quality of the proposed project, (2) availability of funds, and (3) balance among research program areas.

Quality of the Proposed Project

After you receive your summary statement with the priority score, percentile, and critique of your research project, you will have a good idea if there is any chance that you are in a competitive range for funding in this cycle. The percentile is the criterion for the peer-reviewed scientific quality of your research application used in these decisions.

Availability of Funds

Each year the Office on AIDS, NIMH is asked to develop a budget justification and program initiatives, which are submitted to Congress. On the basis of these requests and other considerations, the Office on AIDS receives a budget. Funding decisions for a specific cycle are based on the payline, which is the percentile up to which grants will be paid. The payline is established in each funding cycle by the Director of the Office on AIDS. This number is contingent on many factors (e.g., the number of high-quality applications, available funds, the budget of each grant, etc.).

Balance among Research Areas in Program

Although funding decisions are usually in order of percentile ranking (lowest up to the payline), if your project is in a priority area, you may have a slight advantage if your application received a borderline percentile with respect to the payline for that funding cycle. For example, if X area is a high priority and your grant is in X area but a grant in Y area received a percentile several points lower, you may even your chances of being funded.

The Spending Plan

A spending plan is prepared for each cycle of Council. This is a document prepared by the Office on AIDS to indicate to the NIMH Director which grants are being recommended for payment. After the Institute Director approves the spending plan, it is forwarded to the Budget Office and the Grants Management Branch (GMB) within NIMH. All grants must be on an approved spending plan prior to initiating the payment process.

What Is the Process of Paying Grants?

As stated above, after the Office on AIDS has made the decision about which specific grants will be paid in this funding cycle, a spending plan is prepared and submitted to the Director of NIMH for institutional approval. This approval must be obtained prior to beginning the funding process, which is a careful process among program, grants management, and budget staff that ensures the accuracy of the process. (See Table 1 for the sequence in the funding process.)

What If the IRG Cuts Your Budget?

You should contact your project officer, who will review the summary statement and your application and make a recommendation in writing to the Director, Office on AIDS. If the Director approves it, after consultation and approval of the Scientific Review Administrator (SRA) of your review committee, the Office on AIDS will submit the appropriate paperwork for restoration of funds to the NIMH Council for their consideration.

```
Table 1. The Funding Process

If your grant is in the approved spending plan, the Office on AIDS will contact the appropriate project
officer who will monitor your grant and request that a pay memo be prepared.

The pay memo will be reviewed and approved by the Director, Office on AIDS, and will be forwarded to
the Grants Management Branch, who will double-check the spending plan to confirm that your grant is in
it and will make up an official file.

The pay memo and the official file will then go to a Grants Management Specialist, who will work up the
grant award.

The GMB will then send a draft of the award notice back to the Office on AIDS and to your project
officer to be checked.

After the award notice is checked and returned to the GMB, the final Notice of Grant Award is prepared
and signed by the Chief of the GMB.

The GMB then sends copies of the signed award notice to the NIMH Budget Office for certification that
funds are available.

After receiving funds certification from the NIMH Budget Office, the GMB will mail the Notice of Grant
Award to the grantee institution.

Now you can begin your research project.
```

What If My Grant Did Not Get Referred to NIMH?

If you worked with an NIMH staff person and are responding to an NIMH Program Announcement, you
should send a cover letter with your research application asking for assignment to NIMH. In addition,
indicate in Block 2 of the face page of your application that you are responding to a specific NIMH
Program Announcement or the NIMH AIDS Program. If, despite this, the primary assignment is made to
another Institute, you can still ask that NIMH be listed as the secondary assignment. Then, if you receive
a favorable review and the primary agency does not have the funds to support your grant, NIMH can
request primary assignment to fund the application if you are within the NIMH payline for that funding
cycle. Most Institutes and referral officers are willing to transfer a grant to a secondary Institute if there is
assurance that it will be funded.

How Do I Apply for an Administrative Supplement?

If you find that you need an additional amount of money for a specific activity, you can request an
administrative supplement. Two criteria are important: (1) the amount of money should be "reasonable"

and a small percentage of your grant, and (2) the activity should fall under the original scientific review. If your request does not meet those criteria, you should apply for a competing supplement.

You should communicate your needs to your project officer, who will review the summary statement to be sure that the IRG did not have scientific concerns about that aspect of the original research application. The project officer also reviews your request in light of the progress that you have made in adhering to your timeline and the reasons that additional funds are needed. The project officer then completes a set of forms recommending to the Director, Office on AIDS, that the administrative supplement be paid. If approved by the Director, the necessary paperwork would be forwarded to the GMB to revise the Notice of Grant Award. Information on the administrative supplement is transmitted to the next Council as a courtesy.

Whom Do I Talk to About What?

When you are developing your research application and want to receive critical comments prior to submission, you should talk to a program person. That can be program staff in the Office on AIDS or one of the divisions within the Institute. It is probably beneficial to talk to many persons, because you receive different expertise and perspectives. (See Table 2 for a list of Divisions.)

From the point you submit your research application, you should only speak to the Scientific Review Administrator (SRA) of the assigned review committee about your application. This is the person who will handle the process of scientific review of your application, send you the card within 5 days of the review indicating how your application faired, and ultimately prepare and send your summary statement.

Table 2. NIMH AIDS Program Class Codes and Telephone Numbers

Office of the Director (OD)	301-443-3673
Office on AIDS (AZ-OD)	301-443-7281
Division of Neuroscience and Behavioral Sciences (DNBS)	301-443-3563
Behavioral and Integrative Neuroscience Research (AZ-BN)	301-443-1576
Behavioral, Cognitive, and Social Processes (AZ-BV)	301-443-3942
Molecular and Cellular Neuroscience Research (AZ-MC)	301-443-3948
Division of Clinical and Treatment Research (DCTR)	301-443-5047
Schizophrenia Research Branch (AZ-SZ)	301-443-4707
Mood, Anxiety, and Personality Disorders Research Branch (AZ-AF)	301-443-1636
Mental Disorders of the Aging Branch (AZ-AG)	301-443-1185
Child and Adolescent Disorders Research Branch (AZ-CH)	301-443-5944
Clinical Treatment Research Branch (AZ-TR)	301-443-4527
Division of Epidemiology and Services Research (DESR)	301-443-3648
Basic Prevention and Behavioral Medicine Research Branch (AZ-PB)	301-443-4337
Prevention Research Branch (AZ-PV)	301-443-4283
Services Research Branch (AZ-HS)	301-443-3364
Epidemiology and Psychopathology Research Branch (AZ-EP)	301-443-3774
Violence and Traumatic Stress Research Branch (AZ-VT)	301-443-3728

Technically, you should not begin talking with program staff about your application until you have received the summary statement and the Council has met to review your research application.

When you submit your research application, the referral officer makes a decision about which Institute it should be referred to for review (e.g., if you are referred to NIMH, an MH precedes your grant number). As soon as your application reaches NIMH, it automatically receives the code AZ (AIDS). Then, the OAP assigns a Project Officer based on the area of research of your application.

Although anyone at NIMH is willing to discuss the award process, if you begin with the appropriate program person, your questions may be answered more promptly and accurately.

II

Developing Sections of Your Research Application

Now that you have an overview of NIMH and the review process, this section will provide you with the step-by-step process in the development of your research application. First, Gregory Herek discusses the development of a theoretical framework for your proposed study, which provides a conceptual basis for your research application. Robyn Dawes tells you how to write both a testable and exciting hypothesis that is derivative from your theory. Willo Pequegnat and colleagues suggest ways in which qualitative inquiry can strengthen AIDS research and provide guidance on methods and data analytic strategies. If you are proposing an intervention, Jose Szapocznik and Willo Pequegnat outline the principles to use in designing one that will test your hypotheses. Robert Remien suggests ways in which instruments can be selected and adapted for your study population. If you are considering using immunological measures, you should read the chapter by Janice Kiecolt-Glaser, who provides advice on whether you should use immunological measures in your study and, if so, how they can be integrated into your study. Judith Rabkin reviews critical issues in the protection and confidentiality of human subjects and shares advice on how to facilitate IRB approval. Leonard Mitnick provides advice on how to develop your own résumé and present your staff in a way that strengthens your proposal. H. Gerry Taylor provides guidance on how to develop a data analytical plan and sets of questions to ask yourself to evaluate whether your plan is adequate. Frank Mucha tells you how to develop a budget and financial justification, which is a cross-reference to a research application; he also provides some questions that potential reviewers might ask.

9

Developing a Theoretical Framework and Rationale for a Research Proposal

Gregory Herek

Investigators are drawn to AIDS research because they are concerned about the AIDS epidemic. We often have a special sense of immediacy about the problem because we know and love people with AIDS. Many people who are doing research on AIDS are themselves infected with HIV or belong to a community that has been disproportionately affected by the epidemic.

Our concerns about our loved ones, our communities, and our own well-being can cause us to be impatient. We want an immediate solution to practical problems. If we view theory construction as merely an intellectual exercise, then it can almost seem an intrusion, a distraction from our goal of dealing with the problems people with AIDS are facing now and providing them with help. But if we recognize the centrality of theory to our research endeavor, we will be able to use it as an indispensable tool for making our thinking more rigorous and our findings more meaningful.

All empirical research is based on assumptions. Even purely "descriptive" or "exploratory" studies necessarily involve choices about which variables to observe and at what level of detail. A challenge for researchers planning an empirical study is to make these assumptions explicit, to examine them critically, and to design their investigation in such a way that the resulting data will permit those assumptions to be evaluated and modified appropriately.

This is the process of theory construction. Unfortunately, although all research is based on a theory, many grant proposals lack a well-developed theoretical rationale. The theoretical framework may be implied in the proposal but not formally articulated. Consequently, even though it might be based on a good idea, the application is weak, and it receives a poor scientific review.

The Rationale for Theory Construction and Testing

Theory construction and testing should not be viewed as merely an intellectual exercise (or a nuisance), something to be grafted on to a proposal to make it appear more scientific. Whether or not it is explicitly stated, the researcher's theory guides every aspect of her or his research, from formulation of the initial research question through defining and operationalizing variables to interpreting results. Clearly articulating the theoretical assumptions permits the researcher to strengthen her or his research significantly for at least four reasons.

First, explicitly stating the theoretical assumptions permits them to be evaluated critically. The researcher can identify important omissions or can assess whether undue emphasis is being placed on a particular type of variable or relationship.

Second, the theoretical framework connects the researcher to existing knowledge. Guided by a relevant theory, investigators have a basis for their hypotheses. They can build upon others' work (perhaps in quite different research domains) to identify key variables, including some that may not be intuitively obvious, and to develop hypotheses. When two or more competing methods are available for assessing a particular variable, the theoretical framework may guide the investigator in choosing one of them. A theory can help the researcher prioritize variables and research questions, an important task in an era of limited funding.

Third, articulating the theoretical underpinnings of a research project forces the investigator to address questions of why and how. It permits researchers to move from simply describing a phenomenon observed with a particular sample to generalizing about various aspects of that phenomenon to other groups and situations.

Finally, having a theory helps to identify the limits to those generalizations. Because it explains why and how, a theoretical framework specifies which key variables influence a phenomenon of interest. Consequently, it alerts the researcher to examine how those key variables might differ in disparate populations. Suppose, for example, that an investigator observes that a particular intervention successfully reduces high-risk behavior in a particular sample, and she develops a theory that explains this effect in terms of social support. Based on her theory, she knows that the effectiveness of the intervention with other groups will depend on the nature of social support in those groups and whether it operates in the same way and takes similar forms as in her first sample. Because she has a theory that explains why the intervention was successful, she knows what specific factors might limit the intervention's effectiveness with other groups.

Many existing social science theories have been developed with people from specific backgrounds. Much social psychological theory, for example, was first formulated on the basis of empirical research with samples of white, middle-class, heterosexual college students. Before utilizing these theories, it is always appropriate to consider the factors that might limit their applicability to other populations. Does a particular theory of interpersonal attraction, for example, explain the experiences of gay men in the same way as heterosexual men? Does a cognitive theory of decision making apply equally well to people with high and low levels of formal education? Does a theory of moral judgment explain the experiences of men and women equally well?

Developing a Theoretical Framework

At its simplest level, developing a theoretical framework begins with a research question, proceeds through the identification of key variables and the relationships among them, and results in a plan for observing those variables and relationships empirically. In reality, this is always an iterative process. As the investigator develops hypotheses, new variables often emerge. Questions of operationalization may lead to modification of hypotheses or perhaps even reframing the research question. For the sake of simplicity, however, the different steps in theory construction are presented here in a linear (even if somewhat artificial) sequence, beginning with Table 1.

> ### Table 1. Statement of the Problem
>
> What do you want to do? What questions are you asking in the research? What are your goals?
>
> State your objectives clearly; be specific and concrete (use measurable concepts).
>
> State your specific aims in declarative form.
>
> List your objectives in order of priority, and follow this order throughout the proposal (i.e., use parallel structure throughout the literature review, measurement, data analytic sections, etc.).

Identifying the Phenomenon to Be Understood: The Research Question

The first step in developing a theoretical framework is to pose the research question. A researcher who is interested in high-risk sexual behavior between men, for example, may pose the question simply as, "Why do some men engage in high-risk sexual behavior with other men?" Note that the researcher alternatively could pose the question as, "Why do some men *abstain* from high-risk sexual behavior with other men?" Although both questions focus on high-risk sex between men, they represent decidedly different emphases and are likely to lead the researcher down different paths.

Answering the Research Question: The Rudimentary Theory

The theory is an answer to the research question. Usually, the investigator begins with a fairly simple answer. The question about why some men engage in high-risk sex with other men, for example, might be answered in one of the following ways:

1 Men who engage in high risk sex do so because they lack the social skills necessary for successfully negotiating with their partner.

2 Such men are ignorant of the risks posed by HIV infection or of the ways in which infection can be prevented.

3 Such men do not perceive that social norms support safer sex practices.

4 Such men are sensation seekers and experience risk-taking as powerfully reinforcing.

Obviously, these are only a few possible explanations (which may or may not have a foundation in empirical data). What is important for purposes of the present discussion is that each of them will direct the researcher to emphasize some categories of variables and to de-emphasize others. The first answer/ theory would direct the researcher to examine interpersonal dynamics in sexual encounters; the second focuses on information and knowledge; the third emphasizes cultural norms; and the fourth focuses on personality characteristics and patterns of reinforcement.

Choosing a particular focus is likely to lead the investigator to refine the research question. Depending upon which of the above alternatives is selected, for example, the investigator might reformulate the original question of why some men have high risk sex to, "In what situations do men engage in unsafe sex?" or, "What personality characteristics distinguish men who engage in unsafe sex with other men from those who do not?" or, "How do the social networks of men who have unsafe sex differ from those who do not?"

Identifying Variables of Interest

The research question identifies variables (e.g., constructs that take different values that can be measured). The examples in the previous section, for example, highlight several variables: "frequency of engaging in high risk sexual behavior," "level of negotiating skills during sexual behavior," "level of knowledge about HIV and risk reduction," "perceived social norms," and "level of sensation-seeking." All of these constructs vary, e.g., from low to high. As the investigator refines the theory, the variables may be defined further, and new variables may emerge. "High-risk sexual behavior," for example, may be subdivided into "unprotected anal intercourse," "unprotected oral intercourse with ejaculation," and so on.

It is important that the investigator begin with a conceptual approach to the variables. Unfortunately, investigators sometimes initially identify a measure, a particular sample, or a technology on which they try to build a research application. This approach is reminiscent of the old joke about losing one's keys on the dark sidewalk but looking for them under the streetlight because the light is better. It restricts the investigator from the outset and can prevent her from finding the best answer to the research question. If the researcher recognizes that she is beginning by formulating the variable in terms of "scores on test X," then she is getting ahead of herself.

Specifying Relationships among Variables: Theoretical Hypotheses

Once the variables have been identified, the relationships among them can be specified. The statements that describe these relationships at the conceptual level are the theoretical hypotheses. A theory consists of many theoretical hypotheses. The earlier theory of high-risk sex and negotiations skills, for example, could be used to generate several theoretical hypotheses, including: (1) men with higher levels of verbal skills will be more successful at persuading a partner to practice safer sex; (2) men with lower self-esteem will be more fearful of rejection by a potential partner; (3) men who fear rejection will be less likely to insist on use of condoms during anal intercourse. Note that each hypothesis, as highlighted in Table 2, identifies variables (e.g., level of verbal skills, level of success at persuasion) and a relationship between them.

Operationalizing Variables

Having identified the key variables, it is now time to operationalize them.[1] At this point, the investigator should be as specific and concrete as possible. How will levels of risky sex, self-esteem, or knowledge

---

[1] Editors' note: See also "Instrumentation: Off the Shelf or on Your Own" by Remien, this volume, on selecting and adapting appropriate instruments.

Table 2. Hypotheses[a]

What answers are you proposing for the research question?

A hypothesis describes a relationship between two or more variables.

A variable is a construct (or phenomenon or entity) that can assume different levels (quantities or form); it varies.

In your hypotheses, the variables must be conceptually identifiable and capable of empirical observation.

Similarly, the relationships among the variables (and changes in those relationships) must be conceptually identifiable and operationalizable.

Your hypotheses must be testable (i.e., capable of being falsified).

Your hypotheses may be very specific (as in a laboratory experiment) or general (as in exploratory observational research).

Order your hypotheses to correspond with your stated research questions.

Develop alternative hypotheses whenever possible. In predicting a particular relationship between variables (or explanation for a particular variable), consider alternative explanations, and test for them in your research. Anticipate alternative explanations for your expected results, and include tests for those competing hypotheses.

[a] Editors' note: See also "How Do You Formulate a Testable Exciting Hypothesis?" by Dawes, this volume.

---

about transmission be measured? At this stage, the investigator should consider a wide variety of methods: survey and questionnaire self reports, observation in a naturalistic setting, manipulation of variables in a laboratory experiment, or a naturally occurring field experiment.

Operationalizing the Hypotheses

Once the variables are operationalized, the investigator restates the theoretical hypotheses, substituting the operational variables for the conceptual variables. For example, the theoretical hypothesis, "Men with higher levels of verbal skills will be more successful at persuading a partner to practice safer sex" could be stated operationally as, "Men who score high on the ABC score of verbal ability will report more incidents in which they successfully persuaded a reluctant partner to practice safer sex, using the XYZ questionnaire about sexual experiences in the past 30 days."

Practice in Theory Construction[2]

Pick a phenomenon in which you are interested, and identify a relationship between two or more variables. Develop three general explanations for the relationship by inventing new theories or adapting

[2] This exercise is taken from Stinchcombe, A. L. 1968. *Constructing Social Theories.* New York: Harcourt, Brace, and World, p. 13.

existing ones. Make sure that none of your three theories is known to be false. Identify the key variables that are implicated by each of your theories, and formulate at least three theoretical hypotheses. Try to develop your hypotheses in such a way that they distinguish among the three theories. That is, if the predictions for one theory were supported, the predictions for the other two theories would be negated. Choose appropriate measures for each variable, and operationalize your hypotheses.

Suggestions for Writing the Proposal

The sequence described above is a useful strategy for planning a research proposal. The next challenge is to write the proposal itself. In the section that follows, a series of questions are provided to guide the investigator through the various parts of the proposal.

It is important that the investigator use the theoretical framework to guide the writing of the entire research plan. Theory will guide the researcher in deciding which studies to discuss in the literature review. The theory will help the researcher to select the sample, the methodology, and the techniques for data analysis.

This is not to suggest that an investigator should limit the proposal to a narrow test of a particular theory. Whenever possible, the investigator should design the research in such a way that multiple theories can be tested. In some cases, it will be possible to devise a "critical test," that is, a study that will simultaneously support one theory strongly while refuting one or more competing theories decisively. In other cases, the investigator may take a contextualist approach, that is, conduct a study in which several theories are used, with the goal of specifying under which circumstances or with what populations each one is applicable. In all cases, the investigator should remain open to unanticipated findings, which may lead to the development of a new theory.

Theoretical Framework

Why did you answer your research question as you did? Why did you propose the hypotheses that you did?

- ✔ Clearly outline the theory/model/perspective from which your hypotheses emerge.
- ✔ If the theory is new, clearly explain it in detail, defining all relevant terms and providing examples.
- ✔ If the theory is already established, explain how its application to this topic is appropriate, useful for solving the problem, or will enhance the theory.
- ✔ Explain how you proceeded from a theoretical hypothesis to an empirical hypothesis.
- ✔ A theoretical hypothesis is stated in conceptual, abstract terms, for example: "Perceived discrepancies between personal behavior and attitudes will arouse cognitive dissonance and lead to attitude change."
- ✔ An empirical hypothesis is stated in operational, testable terms, for example: "Subjects who lie about their level of interest in an activity and receive only \$1 will subsequently report greater interest in the activity than will subjects who receive \$20 for lying."

Literature Review

Have these questions been asked before? If so, how have they been answered? Have related questions been asked (e.g., with different populations)? What answers have been obtained?

✔ What are the limitations of past research?

✔ How will you build on past strengths while overcoming limitations? Why is your proposed research worthwhile and necessary?

✔ Your review of previous research should be critical and evaluative of previous research, and it should be synthesizing rather than a comprehensive review.

✔ Demonstrate that you know the literature in this area so well that you can summarize its major themes, findings, strengths, and weaknesses in a small amount of space.

✔ Maintain parallel structure in this section. First, discuss the literature relevant to your first question (and hypothesis); then discuss the literature for your second question, and so on.

Significance

Why are your questions and answers important? Consider four kinds of significance:

✔ Theoretical significance: Contribution to basic knowledge

✔ Methodological significance: Development of new methods or adaptation of old methods

✔ Applied significance: Solution of a specific real-world problem

✔ Social significance: Its benefit to society at large

Method and Design

How will you test your hypotheses and answer your research questions? Be specific and detailed.

✔ Operationalize all variables; justify your leap from theoretical to empirical hypotheses.

✔ Identify the appropriate population from which you will sample, and describe your sampling procedures. Discuss how you will gain access to the sample.

✔ Identify the techniques, methods, and instruments you will use. Specify which tests/scales/questionnaires you will use and which procedures (e.g., content analysis, participant observation, field experiment, survey research). Explain why these are appropriate for your research question.

✔ Describe the procedures you will use to collect data. Tell a story (e.g., from participant's perspective). Two possible strategies for organizing this section: (1) maintain parallel structure, or (2) follow chronological sequence of events as they will happen.

✔ Discuss the reliability and validity of your specific instruments and procedures and of your entire method. Will your results be replicable? Will they be generalizable?

✔ How will you analyze your data? (How will you know whether or not you have answered your research questions?) What statistical methods will be used for each hypothesis? Is your sample sufficiently large to permit the detection of significant differences? (The last question is answered with power analysis)

✔ Construct a timeline or schedule for your research (e.g., month-by-month). How long will the entire project take to complete? [Hint: Keep in mind that you may not be notified of funding until shortly before (and sometimes after!) your proposed startup date. So build in some "slack" at the beginning of the project to permit you to hire and train staff, purchase equipment, finalize subcontracts, and the like.]

✔ Discuss your contingency plans. What is most likely to go wrong, and what will you do if it happens?

10

How Do You Formulate a Testable Exciting Hypothesis?

Robyn Dawes

The first reaction of many reviewers to a research proposal or a journal article is either excitement or boredom. If the proposal is boring, they may approve it, but they are unlikely to vote a high rating. In almost any science a necessary but not sufficient condition for something to be important—which in this context means being fundable, being reportable in good scientific journals, and perhaps having an impact on the field—is that it is exciting. Thus, my first advice about getting proposals funded is to talk to friends in the field about your research idea and evaluate their reactions. Your proposal should elicit excitement; if it does not, you should think more about your ideas.

Using "Not" to Separate Exciting from Boring

What makes a proposal, an idea, or an article boring or exciting? When someone expounds a belief or a theory, excitement is created by the credible possibility that it is *not* true. The greatest compliment to the person proposing the idea is to say, "I do not believe it!" Conversely, a boring hypothesis is one which, although likely to be correct, has no credible alternatives.

Take an example from clinical psychology. A therapist writes that all problems in life follow from low self-esteem. His evidence is, in effect, "I know that because the patients who come to me—who get drunk a lot, who beat up their wives, abuse children, or behave in other terrible ways—do not feel good about themselves." But since few professionals (or other people) hold the opposite belief—that such therapy patients do *not* have low self-esteem—his assertion is boring. Ask yourself: How plausible is it that people would simultaneously do such things, think well of themselves, and enter therapy?

Unfortunately, reading through grant proposals, one often finds similar assertions: "Attitudes will be related to behavior," or "People's use of condoms will be positively related to their estimate of how many people in their social group use condoms." If you insert the word "not" (e.g., "Attitudes will *not* be related to behavior"), it readily becomes apparent that the converse of the assertion is not sensible, and we are dealing with platitudes rather than good, interesting scientific hypotheses.

Believing the Opposite to Be True

In the case of the clinical psychologist's platitude, it would be more interesting to suggest that people's lowering of self-esteem precedes their negative behaviors. This hypothesis is more interesting because the converse has some merit. I could readily believe that lowered self-esteem follows, but does not precede, negative behavior; it seems credible that after people behave badly—for whatever reason—they might start feeling badly about themselves. With an interesting hypothesis you can insert the word "not" and still make sense out of things. However, the fact that the opposite is possible is not sufficient to make a hypothesis exciting; it is also necessary to know something about the phenomenon it describes.

I will give you an example of research about the limitations of clinical judgment that is interesting in just the ways I have mentioned. In many areas concerned with predicting human behavior, an extensive literature supports the generalization that statistical prediction is better than clinical prediction (Dawes et al., 1989). The medical area is ambiguous because it is difficult to give the same input information to a statistical model and to a clinician. But in those cases in which one can, the statistical models tend to perform better.

A very striking example comes from the work of Carroll and his colleagues (1982), who studied the prediction of parole violation. In Pennsylvania, prisoners are released on parole based on an interview conducted after they have served half their time. The parole interviewer knows about three variables that predict parole success or failure: (1) criminal record, (2) behavior in prison, and (3) drug abuse behavior. The interviewer elicits other information and forms an impression of the prisoner. The interviewer then makes a recommendation (which is followed approximately 99 percent of the time) about whether the prisoner should be granted parole. In the Carroll study, the parole interviewer also rated the likelihood that the person would stay out on parole successfully through the end of the period.

Parole success is an unclear concept. There is considerable measurement error because some people might commit crimes but not be caught, while others, who might not have committed a crime, nevertheless come to the attention of the authorities and become incarcerated. However imprecise it is as a measure, parole success correlated to a higher degree with a statistical model based on the three variables (parole candidate's criminal record, number of prison violations, and prior drug use) than with the interviewers' ratings—even though the interviewers were also aware of these variables.

My colleagues and I developed a variant on this type of study. We proposed that a "clinical judge" could make predictions, and instead of building an optimally weighting model or linear model to predict the outcome, we would predict the judge's judgments. If such models could be shown to predict actual outcome when outcome information was available, we could use them when there was no outcome information. We called that "bootstrapping," and it seemed to work (Dawes, 1971).

I then wondered, however, what would happen if we bypassed the clinical judge entirely and instead built an *ad hoc* statistical model based on the same variables. That is, what would happen if we took the variables, oriented them in the right direction, and assigned weights *at random?* To test this somewhat perverse idea, we tried to predict several different types of behavior (e.g., success in graduate school, both in Illinois and Oregon).

It turned out that models with random weights worked as well as the models based on a clinical judge's predictions. They did not do quite as well as the models based on the best weights, but they did much better than the clinicians did in all of five data sets we examined (Dawes & Corrigan, 1974). Our conclusion was that optimal linear models outperform clinical judgment because they are linear models, not because they are optimal.

Now, this work roused some excitement! Because the first journal reviewer did not like the results and remained committed to the idea that the weights of these variables really capture expertise, it took about 1½ years to get the work published in the *Psychological Bulletin*. Before it appeared in print, people would hear about the findings and say, "Oh no, you cannot simply assign weights to variables at random and make as good a prediction as a weighting system based on experts' judgments, and a better prediction than the experts. That's impossible." But they would go to their own data sets and find out that it was true. And that was the greatest compliment. It became a "citation classic" because people simply did not believe it at first. You can make the argument that the real impact of a finding can be assessed by the degree to which people previously believe its opposite to be true.

Testing the "Not" in Research Design

Let us consider now another systematic use of the negative hypothesis testing—the "not"—in research design. A good example is the Salk vaccine experiment in Pittsburgh in 1954, conducted at a time when there was some question about whether and how well the new vaccine would work in preventing polio. The original idea was to test the vaccine by giving it to second graders and observing their rate of polio compared to the rate among first and third graders. But then some statisticians suggested a classical randomized double-blind design. Either give the vaccine or a placebo on a random basis to any second-grade child whose parents wanted them to receive the vaccine. The use of a placebo control group in the study permits estimation of what would have happened if children had *not* gotten the vaccine. (That is the condition that is technically termed a "hypothetical counterfactual.")

In this particular clinical study, randomization proved to be extremely helpful in understanding the vaccine's effect, because the highest rate of polio occurred among those children whose parents wanted them to get the vaccine but who received the placebo (Meier, 1972). If you had simply compared the second graders to the first and third graders, you might have concluded that the vaccine did not work particularly well.

In some instances, if you cannot randomize, you can use a statistical control. Often practical as well as scientific reasons will affect the approach. For example, funding organizations could choose at random the communities they will fund in supporting community-based HIV prevention programs. While that approach would provide a good basis for comparative study, it would be rather unpopular politically.

The policy makers at the Centers for Disease Control (CDC) take a different approach by declaring that they will only fund the best programs. It is extremely difficult to determine the impact of programs they support because it is impossible to know what would have happened if good proposals had not been supported. (Perhaps such areas have other "comparative advantages" as well.)

Alternative Explanations for Findings

People do not always possess rational judgments about the importance of such comparisons in behavior. An example from colleagues' research illustrates an important principle about the spontaneous approaches people use to solve problems (Lichtenstein & Feeney, 1968). People were asked to imagine two cities in wartime: City A and City B. They were asked to judge, based on some distribution, whether a bomb was aimed at City A or City B. It turns out their judgment did not depend on the nature of the distribution. Almost all the subjects assumed that the closer a bomb hit was to A, the more likely it was that it had been aimed at A; the closer it was to B, the more likely it was that B was the target.

But such a judgment is not really rational. A bomb that lands far from A but even farther from B may, for example, be more likely to be aimed at A than is one that lands directly on A. In other words, people did not ask, "How likely are my data given that a particular bomb is aimed at A, versus how likely are they given that it is aimed at B?" Rather, they seem to have asked, "How well does it fit with the idea that it is aimed at A?"

As this bombing problem illustrates, people often base their judgments on whether the evidence seems to fit their ideas. They ignore the possibility that other reasons might account for the same observation, and that other observations are possible, and—most importantly—that many ideas must be considered at the same time. In scientific research, however, you must consider alternative means of explaining your findings. It is easy to get so caught up in the causal relationships between the variables that you end up predicting something that is trivial and thinking the data support it.

Returning to the question of what makes a proposal exciting, I believe that excitement is generated when two or more reasonable hypotheses are compared and research is proposed to show that one of them predicts unusual data better than the other(s). What is most powerful to me as a reviewer of a grant proposal is whether it is going to say, "I believe that these relationships hold, and I am going to test them in such a way that I predict something that others do not predict."

References

Carroll, J., Wiener, R. L., Coates, D., Galegher, J., & Alibrio, J. J. 1982. Evaluation, diagnosis, and prediction in parole decision making. *Law and Society Review 35*, 199–228.

Dawes, R. M. 1971. A case study of graduate admissions: Application of three principles of human decision making. *American Psychologist 26*, 180–188.

Dawes, R. M., & Corrigan, B. 1974. Linear models in decision making. *Psychological Bulletin 81*, 95–106.

Dawes, R. M., Faust, D., & Meehl, P. E. 1989. Clinical versus actuarial judgment. *Science 243:* 1668–1674.

Lichtenstein, S., & Feeney, G. J. 1968. The importance of the data-generating model in probability estimation. *Journal of Organizational Behavior and Human Performance 42*, 62–67.

Meier, P. 1972. The biggest public health experiment ever: 1954 field trial of the Salk poliomyelitis vaccine. In J. M. Tanur, F. Mosteller, W. H. Kruskal, R. F. Link, R. S. Pieters, & G. R. Rising (eds.), *Statistics: A Guide to the Unknown*. San Francisco: Holden-Day, pp. 2–13.

11

Qualitative Inquiry
An Underutilized Strategy in AIDS Research[1]

Willo Pequegnat, Bryan Page, Anselm Strauss, Hortensia Amaro, Paul Goldstein, Richard B. Fritz, Peter Adler, Jeffrey Kelly, and Ali Manwar

Introduction

HIV/AIDS is the third-leading cause of death among adults ages 25 to 44. As of December 31, 1994, there were 441,528 reported cases of AIDS in the U.S.

Currently, the populations most directly affected by the HIV epidemic in the United States are gay and bisexual men and injection drug users (IDUs). However, the number of HIV-infected heterosexual women and adolescents, especially those in urban areas among ethnically diverse groups, is increasing at a rapid rate (Holmes *et al.*, 1990). Each of these populations differs in social culture and behavioral norms. Since health behavior research has historically focused on middle-class populations and because African-Americans and Hispanics have traditionally been underserved in prevention and health research initiatives, little is known about the social context of the populations most imminently threatened by HIV in the second decade of the epidemic (Amaro, 1988).

Because HIV high-risk sexual behaviors in adolescents and adults are interpersonal events involving at least two persons, AIDS prevention requires unprecedented attention to social context factors. Even

---

[1] This chapter is based on a meeting convened by the Office on AIDS, National Institute of Mental Health (NIMH) on May 5–6, 1992, entitled "Qualitative Analysis of Textual and Focus Group Data".

if a vaccine were to be discovered, behavioral approaches would continue to be the crux of prevention campaigns, and currently they are the only way to stem the further spread of HIV and to prevent rapid disease progression. The social pressures, perceptions, and contingencies that establish and maintain high-risk behavior patterns must be understood in order to develop prevention efforts that sustain behavior change (Amaro & Gornemann, 1991; Kelly _et al.,_ 1991a). For example, HIV prevention efforts directed toward inner-city women must recognize that women's HIV risk-reduction efforts may provoke their male partners' violence or withdrawl of fiscal or social support (Worth, 1989, 1990a,b; Ngamathi & Vasquez, 1989).

The goal of this chapter is to encourage qualitative researchers to conduct AIDS research and to encourage collaboration between qualitative and quantitative researchers. This chapter argues that qualitative inquiry is an effective but underused approach to identifying principles of human behavior related to HIV and suggests that AIDS researchers should use this approach in combination with quantitative approaches in well-designed AIDS studies (Kotarba, 1990). After discussing the differences between quantitative and qualitative research, the chapter presents a brief overview of qualitative research and its contribution to AIDS prevention research, as well as potential issues that AIDS researchers will need to address in developing collaborative studies.

Differences between Qualitative and Quantitative Research

Different questions and problems can be optimally explored using the different strategies. Although one can find many commonalities in the approaches, in Table 1 the differences are stressed to highlight the benefits to research from collaboration.

Qualitative Approaches

Qualitative research methods are essential in understanding the values, attitudes, and relationships important to people at high risk for HIV infection in the second decade (Miller _et al.,_ 1990). Disregard of social context factors or the imposition of value systems inconsistent with or counter to the values of a community are likely to produce irrelevant and ineffective interventions with target population (Kelly _et al.,_ 1991b).

Although changing high-risk sexual and drug use behaviors is central to reducing the further spread of HIV infection, the database for designing effective interventions is limited. Sexual behavior and addiction are complex aspects of behavior that are not easily amenable to change (Becker & Joseph, 1987). How people make decisions (or experience coercion) concerning sexual activity, what factors contribute to high-risk patterns with multiple partners, what attitudes and experiences are particularly salient regarding condom use, and how couples negotiate safer sexual practices are all important topics that lend themselves to qualitative study.

Definition of Qualitative Research

Qualitative research constructs a coherent analytic narrative about phenomena in response to a question of interest. The process of gathering information is open and usually inductive, using facts and studying phenomena that are germane to the question (Ridder, 1981). A range of research techniques (e.g., observation, open-ended interviewing, structured interviews and surveys, existing records, and focus groups) can be effective in overcoming biases of memory, self-perception, fear, and mistrust (Grund _et_

Table 1. Differences Between Qualitative and Quantitative Approaches

	Qualitative	Quantitative
Purpose	Describe, understand	Predict causal relationships
Questions	Ask: Why? How?	Test: What?
Logic	Inductive	Deductive
Role of Theory	Broad theoretical models, *post hoc* development of relationships	Theory-driven hypotheses of relationships among variables
Instrumentation	Primarily open and unstructured, face validity	Reliability and validity of instruments established in separate studies
Sampling of Subjects	Availability, purposive, theoretical, snowballing	Exclusion/inclusion criteria established in advance, random assignment, representative control group
Intervention	Observational only, documenting effect of presence in setting	Carefully designed and manipulated by researcher
Data-Gathering Techniques	Immersion, trained observation, in-depth interviewing	Structured interviews, instruments with predetermined response categories
Data Analysis	Verbally descriptive and usually non-numerical	Numerical descriptions and statistics
Role of Researcher	Must establish relationship with subjects	Must be blinded to conditions, standard interaction with subjects

al., 1991). Qualitative research has usually been conducted by researchers trained in anthropology or sociology.

Theoretical Approaches

There are three strategies in formulating a theoretical approach in the design of a qualitative study:

1   *Atheoretical or theory building.* The investigator begins with a single research question, but not *a priori* hypotheses to explore. The investigator intends to build a theory and a set of hypotheses to be tested as the qualitative research progresses and the researcher comes to understand the phenomena under study.

2   *Key research questions.* Based on the researcher's experience, there may be a problem that needs further investigation (e.g., issues in hospice management of endstage AIDS). This problem suggests questions that focus the planned study, even though there may be no stated theory on which they are based nor hypotheses to be tested. This represents a middle ground between having an established theory and beginning with an atheoretical stance.

3   *Theory driven.* The investigator recognizes a theory that may be applicable to the basic research question, and qualitative approaches can be used to examine the questions that emerge from that theory (Glaser, 1978).

Techniques in Qualitative Research

Ethnography and phenomenology are two approaches encompassed under the rubric of qualitative research (Strauss & Corbin, 1990).[2] Our focus is primarily on the potential contribution of ethnography to research on problems associated with HIV infection (Hammersley & Atkinson, 1983). Ethnography has been defined as an "analytical description of behaviors that characterize and distinguish cultures or sociocultural groups." In addition, ethnography describes and analyzes the "knowledge and beliefs that generate and interpret those behaviors" (Walters, 1980, p. 17). Ethnographers establish participant or membership roles in subject populations in order to understand how the subjects perceive the meaning of particular phenomena (Adler & Adler, 1987). While self-report data from surveys have provided information on needle-sharing behavior, these studies do not provide rich contextual descriptions of behaviors that put persons at risk for HIV. Observations by ethnographers about the frequency, conditions, and physical and social milieus of sharing and pooling needles have been essential in understanding the epidemiology of AIDS and in designing effective interventions (Le Compte & Gietz, 1982). Ethnographers have visited shooting galleries, homes, and other places where drug users gather to inject drugs (Watters, 1989) and use crack (Manwar *et al.,* 1994; Williams *et al.,* 1992). They have observed the practices and communications among people who share and pool needles and those who do not and have been able to provide important social and behavioral perspectives on the problems (Guba, 1981; Ouellet *et al.,* 1991).

In addition to direct observation, ethnographers may conduct interviews that are open-ended, structured, or a combination of the two approaches. Well-crafted interviews are a systematic way of gathering data that allows the exploration of observed behavior patterns and can augment what was learned during direct observation. The ethnographer may no longer be viewing the actual behavior, but collecting a detailed account of the behavior.

Because it may be difficult to be present when specific phenomena occur, especially ones that are infrequent, illegal, or private, spending an hour interviewing a research subject who provides descriptions of all recent instances of a specific behavior is cost-effective. Interviews also offer an opportunity to probe into subjects' motivations for engaging in specific behaviors (Goldstein, 1979).

Another useful method of data collection involves examining records that are kept for other reasons, such as official government documents, legal records, or personal diaries. Focus groups offer an additional potent method for collecting qualitative data, one that capitalizes on group interaction to explore the topic in greater depth (Morgan, 1988). This method can also be used when time or resource limitations preclude individual interviews. Focus groups can provide early impressions of a target population, assist in developing interview protocols, facilitate the assessment of prevention materials, delineate behavior under different policies, and validate and/or elaborate on information gathered by other means. While focus groups may meet only one time, depending on the research question, there may be advantages to convening them several times to explore changes over time.

Settings for Qualitative Research

Traditionally, behavioral scientists have studied behaviors within traditional institutions (e.g., college campuses, mental hospitals, community mental health facilities). However, populations in which HIV infection is now rapidly increasing may not be reached effectively through these institutions. Such people may be suspicious of institutions and may not have a tradition of discussing personal or family matters with strangers. Standard instruments with good psychometric properties may seem foreign or unrelated to their personal experiences.

---

[2] For descriptions of these approaches, the reader should consult N. Denzin & Y. Lincoln, eds. 1993. *Handbook on Qualitative Research.* Newbury Park, CA: Sage.

To reach these populations, researchers must move beyond simply studying institutionally accessible populations and seek alternative places and methods for studying persons at risk (Broadhead & Fox, 1990; Kotarba, 1990). Through regular observation of behavior and interactive questioning about its meaning within a sociocultural context, a qualitative strategy may allow description of patterns of behavior that are otherwise private (Des Jarlais *et al.*, 1986; Polsky, 1967). Recently ethnographers have been making more use of ethnographic field stations, such as store fronts or apartments in housing projects. These research outposts in communities of interest facilitate the conduct of observation, interviewing, and focus groups. They also provide a stable base of operations for the researchers and enhance the continuity of researcher and subject relationships (Goldstein *et al.* 1990).

Sampling Techniques

Qualitative research uses a number of sampling techniques to gain access to subjects (Bernard, 1988). Using an availability sampling strategy, the researcher identifies settings where people who are knowledgeable about the topic are found. For example, a researcher interested in studying pickup patterns of single persons might go to singles bars and interview whoever is there (Stall *et al.*, 1990). Similarly, if interested in drug overdose, the researcher might stake out an emergency room of an urban hospital. A snowballing strategy permits the researcher to trace networks of informal relations to expand the number of people interviewed whose life experience is relevant to questions under study. By contrast, a purposive or targeted sampling strategy involves establishing, in advance, geographic, age, or other criteria related to the research question. The researcher then approaches multiple networks in order to identify persons to interview who meet those criteria. Theoretical sampling is akin to targeted sampling, but the criteria are derived from initial inquiries rather than *a priori*, and it is based on concepts that have demonstrated relevance to the emerging theory.

Data Analytic Approaches

The collection of qualitative data usually results in large amounts of material—interviews, field notes, and transcripts of focus group discussions. The researcher must choose the mode of analysis that will achieve the goals of the research (Miles & Huberman, 1984; Strauss, 1987). A quantitative researcher who intends to collaborate with a qualitative researcher should be alert to the different modes of data analysis, since researchers are not equally skilled (Fritz, 1988).

Ethnographic data by their very nature require an interpretation; meaning must be deciphered from descriptions of action, ritual, belief, symbol, or other social fact (Blumer, 1969; Denzin, 1969, 1989). The same meaning of an informant's answer to a question will depend upon who said it and how, when, and in what context it was said (Goodenough, 1970). There are different ways that texts can be analyzed to understand the culture or subculture under investigation (Clifford & Marcus, 1986; Garfinkel, 1967; Marcus & Cushman, 1982).

Description When the research is aimed at communicating the subjects' viewpoints directly, a descriptive mode is traditionally used (Spradley, 1980). This technique is valuable when the culture of the study population is different from the culture of the intended readers of the research (Farmer, 1990). Description of behaviors, events, and social context can be most powerful when the researcher includes direct quotations from the interviewees or observed subjects. Observations at a shooting gallery might describe the events at different times of the day (e.g., Who was there? What was going on? What did they say?). Descriptions can stand alone or be used in conjunction with other modes of qualitative data analysis. While this mode of analysis can be complex in the selection and arrangement of materials, it is not at a high level of abstraction.

Theme Analysis Another mode of analysis that reduces the data to an orderly interpretation is called theme analysis. Repeated statements or events that point to a common thread or theme are identified in the interviews or field notes (Lofland & Lofland, 1984; Jorgensen, 1989). For example, Hispanic women frequently report that "machismo" and power imbalance between men and women create barriers to negotiating safer sex and condom use (Amaro & Gornemann, 1992). Another theme might be the fact that economic survival or crime in the streets has more immediacy to poor people than does AIDS prevention. Theme analysis can vary in the amount and explicitness of the explanation of the themes and their implications.

Analysis of Social or Cultural Patterns Theme analysis can merge into analysis of patterns that provide a social context for the themes. Pattern analysis can become complex, since the research is relating subpatterns to each other and to an overall pattern structure. For example, the study of husbands' abuse of their wives revealed that women's reports of the abuse were often discounted by police and social workers (Loseke, 1992). In explaining this discounting, Lempert (1992) reviewed the available literature on those professions and observed that both the nature of police work and the professional experiences of social workers mitigated serious consideration of the women's "complaints." A more elaborate study might have interviewed the police and social workers themselves.

The researcher also discussed why many of the women could not quickly leave their marital relationships, relating this inaction to their upbringing as young women and their expectations of marriage. These conclusions were reached through intensive interviewing of the women and by attending and observing many meetings of a support group of abused wives.

The numerous quantitative studies of spouse abuse had not captured the process whereby women finally recognized themselves as abused and acted. This form of qualitative analysis is essential in understanding the decision-making process in AIDS prevention behaviors (e.g., how partners negotiate safer sexual practices).

Theoretical Analysis Qualitative data are rich in potential for developing as well as extending theory. Recently, qualitative researchers have set forth explicit procedures for developing theory efficiently and at different levels of abstraction (Strauss & Corbin, 1990). This work requires elaborate coding, the relating of categories in a variety of ways, and their integration into an overall theoretical statement, framework, or model (Bolton, 1992). The analysis of patterns often entails implicit theory development, which can become more explicit and elaborate (Douglas, 1976). Contemporary qualitative researchers are more likely to develop theory from their data and then link it with existing theory rather than use qualitative data to verify existing theory. Depending on the modes of data analysis, different software packages may be appropriate (Fritz, 1988). Descriptive analysis requires software programs that provide quick and easy retrieval of quotations and descriptive items. Pattern analysis and theoretical analysis, by contrast, require programming for sorting and relating items. Tesch (1989, 1991) notes that only a few programs address the requirements of theorizing, but programs are under development to aid in the elaborate work of relating concepts.

Criteria for Evaluating Qualitative Studies

Qualitative researchers do not use the same tests of reliability and validity as quantitative researchers do (Kvale, 1989). Rather, qualitative researchers invoke a set of criteria for judging the scientific rigor of their work. In evaluating an ethnography, the researcher must demonstrate either a role in the setting or some means of access that permits an accurate portrait of the people (Douglas, 1976; Johnson, 1975). The extent to which a research project facilitates development of these complex roles between the researcher and subject is one measurement of its success (Adler & Adler, 1987).

Strauss and Corbin (1990) provide guidance on what descriptions are required to permit others to evaluate research conducted using grounded theory. These criteria can also be used to evaluate whether the concepts emerged from the data in other approaches to qualitative research: (1) an explicit description of the research questions, (2) the method and rationale for sample selection, (3) the analytic categories that emerged, (4) the actions and events that pointed to these categories, and (5) the hypotheses that might be generated. Although the nomenclature comes from grounded theory, the criteria can be translated into other modes of qualitative research (Glaser & Strauss, 1967). Instead of analytic categories, ethnographers may have other names for significant units of analysis (e.g., "concepts" may become "values").

Data analysis should result in an internally coherent conceptual framework that allows the reader to judge the validity and accuracy of the conclusions. The reader should derive new insights or unique illustrations of some taken-for-granted theory that must extend, modify, or refute extant knowledge (Davis, 1971).

Overview of Qualitative Approaches in AIDS Research

The following section reviews some areas in which qualitative research has made a contribution to AIDS research and suggests other possible directions:

1. Providing different interpretation of data
2. Accessing hard-to-reach populations
3. Collecting different data
4. Improving flexibility of the data-gathering process
5. Differentiating ethnic groups
6. Operationalizing variables
7. Developing instruments
8. Expanding technology transfer
9. Evaluating policy and interventions

Providing Different Interpretation of Data

While quantitative and qualitative researchers may use some of the same techniques, differences in the way the data are analyzed may yield different results. Ethnographic methods may be used to collect data that can be quantified (e.g., frequency and amount of drugs used), which permits analytic techniques such as descriptive statistics or time series analysis (Goldstein *et al.* 1991; Fendrich *et al.* 1992). In addition, qualitative data analysis can provide another approach to extracting useful information from the data.

The use of qualitative techniques can aid in interpreting the findings when anomalous trends or differences between populations are observed in small studies or large-scale surveys. Ethnographers' direct experiences with research subjects and phenomena permit conceptualization of discrete events as patterns of behavior. If there is a contradiction between what people are saying and what they are doing, qualitative researchers can provide some insights.

Using qualitative methods, Carrier (1989) was able to identify subtle but real differences in definition of roles in same-gender sexual behavior among Mexican men. In a population of Mexican men in northern California, Alonso and Koreck (1989) confirmed this, finding that the insertive sexual partner is not viewed as homosexual. Gay-oriented prevention messages may therefore not be effective in reaching these men.

Accessing Hard-to-Reach Populations

Eliciting details about sexual behaviors or illicit drug use poses critical challenges to the researcher. Even in populations where surveys are commonplace and there is little fear of breaching confidentiality, these topics can present difficulties. In populations unaccustomed to survey inquiries, these difficulties are compounded. Qualitative methods, and specifically ethnographic methods, can assist researchers in gathering information that would otherwise be inaccessible (Des Jarlais & Friedman, 1990).

Collecting Different Data

In many areas of HIV research, qualitative methods could provide important insights into a range of topics relevant to prevention and intervention (Adler, 1985, 1990a; Campbell, 1991). Ethnographic methods could be used, for example, to investigate the use and disposition of needles distributed through needle-exchange programs (Stimson, 1989). Ethnographic research could be useful in understanding the underlying causes of the erosion of safer sex practices among gay men (Kelly *et al.*, 1991a; Martin, 1987; Wilkelstein *et al.*, 1987). It could also be used to develop data on stigma or personal identity in order to design strategies that might sustain HIV avoidance behaviors (Kowalewski, 1988; Sandstrom, 1990).

For example, in two studies of the relationship between HIV infection and injection drug use, investigators administered structured interviews on needle-use patterns (in Denver, Koester, 1989; in Miami, Chitwood *et al.*, 1990; Page *et al.*, 1990a,b,c). While these interviews included specific questions on sharing or pooling of needles, cookers (vessels in which injectable drugs are mixed and/or heated to liquify them), and cottons (cotton balls used to filter liquid drawn into the syringe), even these exhaustive inquiries would have missed an area of risk behavior. In both studies, however, the investigators also conducted direct observations in an injection safe house or shooting gallery. These studies permitted them to observe that the rinse water also represented a risk. In Denver, the observer noticed that rinse water became increasingly pink because users were injecting themselves with syringes that, although previously rinsed with bleach, made contact with shared water before injection. In Miami, the ethnographers found that houses provided "clean" and "dirty" water (one for mixing drugs in the cooker and the other for rinsing the syringe). Injectors used a common jar of dirty water to rinse their syringes and drew from the clean jar to mix their drugs, which, because of common usage, were potentially HIV-infected.

Another study in a shooting gallery revealed the critical role of the person who supervises its activity in influencing clients' needle-cleaning behavior (Page, 1990). These findings suggested that keeping the "house man" interested and involved in supplying bleach and clean water to clients is critical in maintaining clients' risk-reduction behavior (Page *et al.*, 1990b).

The use of in-depth interviews, a method often used in qualitative research, was critical in identifying severe gaps in HIV prevention knowledge and practice among male clients of female street prostitutes (Leonard, 1987). These findings suggest that clients present a more serious threat to the public health than prostitutes, because clients not only lack knowledge about HIV risk but have multiple liaisons both with prostitutes and with women not engaged in prostitution (Worth, 1989).

Limited research indicates that the riskiness of people's sexual practices tend to be congruent with perceived norms concerning the social acceptability of safer sexual practices (Carrier & Bolton, 1992; Kelly *et al.*, 1990). While this is potentially one of the most promising foci for community-level AIDS prevention approaches, it has not yet been carefully studied. Qualitative research methods can elucidate patterns of social influence over risk-taking, identify the most important sources of this influence, and suggest strategies for redefining social and peer norms to reinforce risk avoidance (Katz *et al.* 1963).

Mixed-discipline, -gender, and -ethnic teams can obtain data that might not be available to individual researchers with a single approach. Regular discussions at team meetings can provide a cross-check on observations and opinions and can provide support for handling the stress associated with field research. Involving people from the study population in deliberations of the research team can clarify findings and ensure recruitment and retention of research subjects from the community.

Improving Flexibility of the Data Collection Process

An advantage of qualitative research is the ability to reformulate and refine research questions as the study progresses in order to pursue promising avenues of inquiry. Because quantitative surveys usually investigate only predetermined issues, they may not offer an effective way to discover previously unnoticed or newly emergent issues. Skepticism about the latest qualitative findings is built into the investigator's *a priori* research design to check emerging data with previous findings (Adler, 1990b). This strategy would not be permitted under the scientific tenets of quantitative research.

For example, if an epidemiological study based on a hospital's outpatient data identified a relationship between gang membership and HIV seropositivity, a qualitative study designed to explain this phenomenon might focus on the behavior of youths in gangs. The initial question might be: "What behaviors in the context of gang activities carry risk of HIV infection?" The study population would then be members of a youth street gang in the hospital's catchment area.

Observing gang activities may reveal that the research questions are inappropriate or may document that risk behaviors do not occur during gang activities. To remedy this the investigator might shift from natural observations alone to open-ended questions and, eventually, to examination of non-gang behaviors. If further study documents that high-risk behaviors are practiced elsewhere but maintained by gang membership, the gang would be confirmed as the appropriate point of intervention.

Differentiating Ethnic Groups

Regional origin or SES (social and economic status) within an ethnic group may predict more about behavior than simply group membership. For example, Asian Americans, Japanese, Koreans, Taiwanese, and Chinese have distinct cultures and behavioral expectations that may differ as much from one another as from mainstream U.S. culture. Qualitative research methods can provide data that clarify these differences.

Operationaling Variables

In addition to explaining and elaborating quantitative trends, ethnographers contribute to increasing the utility and standardization of functional definitions of key variables (e.g., what is a "shooting gallery," "smokehouse," or drug dealer?).

Developing Instruments

Ethnographers can contribute to the formulation of all aspects of surveys. For example, their sensitivity to the use of language and argot can aid in phrasing questions to elicit valid data (Cicourel, 1964). Drug users often respond in the negative to questions about "use" of certain drugs because "use" implies dependence; however, they might respond in the affirmative to questions about whether they have "tried" the drugs. Also, in Chicago, questions about "crack" use may elicit negative responses because locally that substance is called "rock," or "ready-rock," and some users believe that it is different from crack.

Expanding Technology Transfer

Behavioral scientists are often employed in university settings, where performance standards differ from those of direct service providers. Researchers do not necessarily conduct studies that are useful for answering the questions that health care workers or service providers have about how to intervene with different populations. Cross-sectional studies that collect data only on the frequency of behaviors and knowledge of risk may not capture the rich context in which behaviors occur and are reinforced. The results may not translate into information upon which effective interventions can be designed nor advice be provided to service providers on appropriate prevention strategies.

Early in the AIDS epidemic knowledge, attitude, and behavior (KAB) studies of different populations were important. These studies identified gaps in people's understanding about HIV and provided critical information on the risk behaviors in which people were engaging. The data provided guidance on developing interventions and educational programs for groups that were motivated to change. This approach did not, however, provide a fertile data set upon which to develop specific prevention programs tailored to specific groups on the basis of where people gained knowledge of HIV, how their attitudes were formed, and how the behaviors took place. Qualitative studies that describe and analyze these contexts and processes represent a critical factor in translating findings into practice.

Another area in which research studies have provided important findings but little guidance to health care workers concerns the assessment of cognitive dysfunction. While these data are intrinsically important and have provided an understanding of the problems associated with HIV infection of the central nervous system (CNS), these studies have not taken the next step to link this assessment data with everyday functioning. If HIV-infected persons have compromised speed of information processing, what does this mean about their lifestyle, their daily life, and the treatments or supportive interventions that might be developed to support independent living as long as possible?

Evaluating Policy and Interventions

Another benefit to AIDS research that can result from collaboration is in the evaluation of policies and interventions. Ethnographers are often in an advantageous position to provide expert advice on policy development and to study the impact of policies, legislation, or interventions on target populations (Broadhead & Fox, 1990; Campbell, 1991; Des Jarlais & Friedman, 1990). They may be part of an early warning system (e.g., Drug Alert Warning Network [DAWN] and Drug Use Forecast [DUF])[3] or provide insight into newly emerging social problems (e.g., the apparent current resurgence in heroin use) that are relevant to the AIDS epidemic. They can provide important information on how subgroups may be negatively affected by a policy or how a media campaign may be misdirected (Inciardi, 1990). For

---

[3] The National Institute on Drug Abuse (NIDA) supports DAWN to identify drug use patterns in hospital emergency rooms, and the National Institute of Justice (NIJ) supports DUF to track recent arrestees.

example, the effect of a campaign to inform men of the dangers of unprotected sex with prostitutes resulted in many of them having unprotected sexual relationships with younger inexperienced women rather than using condoms (Bledsoe, 1990).

Integrating Qualitative and Quantitative Strategies

Developing collaborative research efforts often requires overcoming long-held misconceptions and prejudices. Quantitative researchers have been willing to use qualitative approaches as exploratory strategies but rely solely on quantitative methods to provide confirmatory data. However, qualitative research can also be effective when combined with a quantitative approach (Miles, 1983), but it is critical that the two strategies be well integrated in the study design.

When embarking on a collaboration, some practical considerations need to be addressed prior to the proposal writing:

1 Organizational plan and role assignments

2 Provision for adequate level of administration

3 Training and supervision of ethnographers

4 Tension between observation and intervention

Organizational Plan and Role Assignments

Successful collaboration requires an organizational plan that clearly specifies role assignments that are tied to specific research objectives (Douglas, 1976). Role assignments should be based on the individual's expertise and experience. Otherwise, potentially good specific aims may not be achieved because of unclear or conflicting expectations (e.g., amount of time field research requires, lack of recognition for contribution).

Provision for Adequate Level of Administration

The study design should make adequate provision of time and staffing for administrative duties. Ethnographers cannot both work in the field collecting data and handle all the administrative problems in a field site (e.g., managing outreach workers' schedules, handling field station crises unrelated to data collection).

Training and Supervision of Ethnographers

A major problem in conducting qualitative research is the shortage of well-trained qualitative researchers. There is clearly a need for more skilled ethnographers in the field of AIDS research and, consequently, for training programs that will produce them, especially African-American, Hispanic, and Native American ethnographers. As the epidemic of HIV infection is changing, AIDS research is increasingly conducted in culturally diverse communities. This research will have greater validity and acceptability when the data collection and interpretation are conducted by investigators who are well prepared to understand the culture and worldview of the subjects (Lonner & Berry, 1986).

Tension between Observation and Intervention

AIDS research projects, especially those tied to intervention efforts, must address the inevitable tensions between the objectives of observation and behavior change (Broadhead & Fox, 1990). Ethnographers do not traditionally implement interventions, but AIDS projects are often designed to persuade IDUs to cease injection or to adopt safer drug-using techniques (e.g., use of bleach) or to convince people to practice abstinence or to adopt safer sex techniques (e.g., use of condoms). Researchers using a qualitative approach try to be nonjudgmental when relating to subjects, but this posture is not easy to maintain in projects devoted to encouraging AIDS-risk reduction.

Future Directions

Qualitative research has been important in revealing key features of behaviors that may not have been identified using strictly quantitative methods. Beyond simply offering access to otherwise inaccessible populations and behaviors, ethnographic studies deepen and elaborate many topics relevant to the AIDS epidemic (Johnson, 1990). Future areas of research that might be effectively pursued include family responses to HIV in relation to prevention efforts, values underlying the use of hypodermic paraphernalia among IDUs, sexual practices of adolescents in relation to their self-concept and way of life, features of individuals' quality of life that guide their choices for medical management of HIV infection and AIDS, and the role of peers in influencing adolescent risk behavior.

People respond to the threat of HIV infection or the fact of HIV infection in qualitatively definable ways. We now need to focus the attention of competent qualitative analysts on how people respond to HIV infection or the threat of infection in order to prevent further spread of infection among the uninfected and to prevent undue suffering among the already infected. The behavioral choices that people make in the face of the AIDS epidemic raise complex questions. To answer them, we must take time to understand those at risk by using qualitative inquiry to design culturally competent prevention programs.

References

Adler, P. A. 1985. *Wheeling and Dealing*. New York: Columbia University Press.

Adler, P. A. 1990a. Ethnographic research on hidden populations: Penetrating the drug world. In: E. Y. Lambert, ed., *The Collection and Interpretation of Data from Hidden Populations*. Rockville, MD: National Institute on Drug Abuse, Research Monograph Number 98, pp. 96–112.

Adler, P. 1990b. Requirements for inductive analysis. In: E. Y. Lambert, ed., *The Collection and Interpretation of Data from Hidden Populations*. Rockville, MD: National Institute on Drug Abuse, Research Monograph Number 98, pp. 44–58.

Adler, P. A., & Adler, P. 1987. *Membership Roles in Field Research*. Newbury Park, CA: Sage.

Alonso, A. M., & Koreck, M. T. 1989. Silences: Hispanics, AIDS, and sexual practices. *Differences 1:* 101–124.

Amaro, H. 1988. Considerations for prevention of HIV infection among Hispanic women. *Psychology of Women Quarterly 12:* 429–443.

Amaro, H., & Gornemann, I. 1991. Health care utilization for sexually transmitted diseases: Influence of patient and provider characteristics. In: A. O. Sergi, J. Warerheit, and K. K. Holmes eds., *Research Issues in Human Behavior and Sexually Transmitted Diseases in the AIDS Era*. Washington, DC: American Society of Microbiology, pp. 140–160.

Amaro, H., & Gornemann, I. 1992. HIV/AIDS related attitudes, beliefs and behaviors among hispanics in the U.S. northeast and Puerto Rico. Report prepared for the Northeast & Hispanic AIDS Coalition. Boston University School of Public Health, Boston, MA.

Becker, M., & Joseph, J. 1987. AIDS and behavioral change in risk reduction: A review. *American Journal of Public Health 78:* 394–410.

Bernard, H. R. 1988. *Research Methods in Cultural Anthropology*. Newbury Park, CA: Sage.

Bledsoe, C. 1990. The politics of AIDS and condoms for stable heterosexual relations in Africa: Recent evidence from the local print media. In: W. P. Handwerker, ed., *Births and Power: The Politics of Reproduction*. Boulder, CO: Westview Press, pp. 197–223.

Blumer, H. 1969. *Symbolic Interactionism*. Englewood Cliffs, NJ: Prentice-Hall.

Bolton, R. 1992. AIDS and promiscuity: Muddles in the models of HIV prevention. In: R. Bolton & M. Singer, eds., *Rethinking AIDS Prevention: Cultural Approaches*, Philadelphia: Gordon and Breach Science Publishers; pp. 7–85.

Broadhead, R. S., & Fox, K. 1990. Takin' it to the streets: AIDS outreach as ethnography. *Journal of Contemporary Ethnography 19:* 322–348.

Campbell, C. A. 1991. Prostitution, AIDS, and preventive health behavior. *Social Science and Medicine 32:* 1367–1378.

Carrier, J. M. 1989. Sexual behavior and the spread of AIDS in Mexico. *Medical Anthropology 10:* 129–142.

Carrier, J., & Bolton, R. 1992. Anthropological perspectives on sexuality and HIV prevention. *Annual Review of Sex Research 2:* 49–75.

Centers for Disease Control. 1994. *Mortality and Mobidity Weekly Report: The Second 100,000 Cases of AIDS*. Atlanta, GA: Centers for Disease Control.

Chitwood, D. D., McCoy, C. B., Inciardi, J. A., McBride, D. C., Comerford, M. A., Trapido, E., McCoy, V., Page, J. B., Griffin, J., Fletcher, M. A., & Ashman, M. A. 1990. HIV seropositivity of needles from shooting galleries in South Florida. *American Journal of Public Health 80:* 150–152.

Cicourel, A. 1964. *Method and Measurement in Sociology*. New York: Free Press.

Clifford, J., & Marcus, G., 1986. *Writing Culture*. Berkeley, CA: University of California Press.

Davis, M. 1971. That's interesting! Toward a phenomenology of sociology and a sociology of phenomenology. *Philosophy of Social Science 1:* 309–344.

Denzin, N. K. 1969. Symbolic interactionism and ethnomethodology: A proposed synthesis. *American Sociological Review 34:* 922–934.

Denzin, N. K. 1989. *The Research Act*. Englewood Cliffs, NJ: Prentice-Hall.

Denzin, N. K., & Lincoln, Y., eds., 1993. *Handbook on Qualitative Research*. Newbury Park, CA: Sage.

Des Jarlais, D. C., Friedman, S. R., & Strug, D. 1986. AIDS and needle sharing within the IV-drug use subculture. In: D. A. Feldman & T. M. Johnson, eds., *Social Dimensions of AIDS: Method and Theory*. New York: Praeger, pp. 111–125.

Des Jarlais, D. C., & Friedman, S. R. 1990. "Shooting galleries" and AIDS: Infection probabilities and "tough" policies. *American Journal of Public Health 80:* 142–144.

Douglas, J. D. 1976. *Investigative Social Research*. Beverly Hills, CA: Sage.

Farmer, P. 1990. Sending sickness: Sorcery, politics, and changing concepts of AIDS in rural Haiti. *Medical Anthropology Quarterly 4(1):* 6–27.

Fendrich, M., Goldstein, P. J., Tarshish, G., & Bellucci, P. A. 1992. Longitudinal measurement of substance use in ethnography samples. *Journal of Community Psychology 20:* 326–342.

Fritz, R. B. 1988. Computer analysis of qualitative data. Collection and interpretation of data for hidden populations: Qualitative research designs. NIDA Technical Review, Rockville, MD.

Garfinkel, H. 1967. *Studies in Ethnomethodology*. Englewood Cliffs, NJ: Prentice-Hall.

Glaser, B., & Strauss, A. 1967. *The Discovery of Grounded Theory*. Chicago: Aldine.

Glaser, B. 1978. *Theoretical Sensitivity*. Mill Valley, CA: Sociology Press.

Goldstein, P. J. 1979. *Prostitution and Drugs*. Lexington, MA.: Lexington Books.

Goldstein, P. J., Spunt, B. J., Miller, T., & Bellucci, P. A. 1990. Ethnography field stations. In: E. Y. Lambert, ed., *The Collection and Interpretation of Data from Hidden Populations*. Rockville, MD: National Institute on Drug Abuse, Research Monograph Number 98, pp. 80–95.

Goldstein, P. J., Bellucci, P. A., Spunt, B. J., & Miller, T. 1991. Volume of cocaine and violence: A comparison between men and women. *Journal of Drug Issues 21(2):* 345–367.

Goodenough, W. H. 1970. Componential analysis and the study of meaning. *Language 32:* 195–218.

Grund, J. C. P., Kaplan, C. D., & Adriaans, N. F. P. 1991. Needle sharing in the Netherlands: An ethnographic analysis. *American Journal of Public Health 81:* 1602–1607.

Guba, E. G. 1981. Criteria for assessing the trustworthiness of naturalistic inquiry. *Educational Communication and Technology–A Journal of Theory 30:* 233–252.

Hammersley, M., & Atkinson, P. 1983. *Ethnography: Principles in Practice*. New York: Travistock.

Holmes, K. K., Karon, J. M., & Kreiss, J. 1990. The increasing frequency of heterosexually acquired AIDS in the United States, 1983–88. *American Journal of Public Health 80(7):* 858–863.

Inciardi, J. A. 1990. Federal efforts to control the spread of HIV and AIDS among IV drug use. *American Behavioral Scientist 33:* 408–18.

Johnson, J. 1990. Ethnopharmocology: An interdisciplinary approach to the study of intravenous drug use and HIV. *Journal of Contemporary Ethnography 17:* 349–369.

Johnson, J. M. 1975. *Doing Field Research.* New York: Free Press.

Jorgensen, D. L. 1989. *Participant Observation.* Newbury Park, CA: Sage.

Katz, E., Levin, M. L., & Hamilton, H. 1963. Traditons of research on the diffusion of innovation. *American Sociological Review 28:* 237–252.

Kelly, J. A., St. Lawrence, J. S., Brasfield, T. L., Lemke, A., Amidei, T., Roffman, R. E., Hood, H. V., Smith, J. E., Kilgore, H., & McNeill, C. 1990. Psychological factors that predict AIDS high-risk versus AIDS precautionary behavior. *Journal of Consulting and Clinical Psychology 58:* 117–120.

Kelly, J. A., Kalichman, S. C., Kauth, M. K., Kilgore, H. G., Hood, H. V., Campos, P. E., Rao, S. M., Brasfield, T. L., & St. Lawrence, J. S. 1991a. Situational factors associated with AIDS risk behavioral lapses and coping strategies used by gay men who successfully avoid lapses. *American Journal of Public Health 81:* 1335–1338.

Kelly, J. A., St. Lawrence, J. S., Diaz, Y. E., Stevenson, L. Y., Hauth, A. C., Brasfield, T. L., Kalichman, S. C., Smith, J. E., & Andrew, M. E. 1991b. HIV risk behavior reduction following intervention with key opinion leaders of population: An experimental analysis. *American Journal of Public Health 81:* 168–171.

Koester, S. 1989. The risk of HIV transmission from sharing water, drug-mixing containers, and cotton filters among intravenous drug users. Unpublished manuscript, University of Colorado School of Medicine, Boulder, CO.

Kotarba, J. A. 1990. Ethnography and AIDS: Returning to the streets. *Journal of Contemporary Ethnography 19:* 259–270.

Kowalewski, M. 1988. Double stigma and boundary maintenance: How gay men deal with AIDS. *Journal of Contemporary Ethnography 17:* 211–228.

Kvale, S., ed. 1989. *Issues of Validity in Qualitative Research.* Lund, Sweden: Studenlitteratur.

Le Compte, N., & Gietz, J. 1982. Problems of reliability and validity in ethnographic research. *Review of Educational Research 52:* 31–60.

Lempert, L. 1992. The crucible: Violence, help-seeking, and abused women's transformations of self. Doctoral dissertation presented to the Department of Social and Behavioral Sciences, University of California at San Francisco.

Leonard, T. L. 1987. Male clients of female street prostitutes: Unseen partners in sexual disease transmission. *Medical Anthropology Quarterly 4(1):* 41–55.

Lofland, J., & Lofland, L. 1984. *Analyzing Social Settings.* Belmont, CA: Wadsworth.

Lonner, W. J., & Berry, J. W. 1986. *Field Methods in Cross-Cultural Research.* Beverly Hills, CA: Sage.

Loseke, D. R. 1992. *The Battered Woman and Shelters: The Social Construction of Wife Abuse.* Albany, NY: State University of New York Press.

Manwar, A., Johnson, B. D., & Dunlop, E. 1994. Qualitative data analysis with hypertext: A case of New York City crack dealers. *Qualitative Sociology 17:* 283–291.

Marcus, G. E., & Cushman, D. 1982. Ethnographies as texts. *Annual Review of Anthropology 11:* 25–69.

Martin, J. L. 1987. The impact of AIDS on gay male sexual behavior in New York City. *American Journal of Public Health 77:* 578–581.

Miles, M. 1983. Mixing qualitative and quantitative methods: Triangulation in action. In: J. Van Maanen, ed., *Qualitative Methodology* (pp. 143–161). Beverly Hills, CA: Sage.

Miles, M., & Huberman, A. 1984. *Qualitative Data Analysis.* Beverly Hills, CA: Sage.

Miller, H. G., Turner, C. F., & Moses, L. I., eds. 1990. *AIDS: The Second Decade.* Washington, D. C.: National Academy Press.

Morgan, D. L. 1988. *Focus Groups as Qualitative Research.* Newbury Park, CA: Sage.

Nyamathi, A., & Vasquez, R. 1989. Impact of poverty, homelessness, and drugs on Hispanic women at risk for HIV infection. *Hispanic Journal of Behavioral Sciences 11(4):* 299–314.

Ouellet, L., Jimenez, A., Johnson, W., & Wiebel, W. 1991. Shooting galleries and HIV disease: Variations in places for injecting illicit drugs. *Crime and Delinquency 27(1):* 64–85.

Page, J. B. 1990. Shooting scenarios and risk of HIV infection. *American Behavioral Scientist 33:* 478–490.

Page, J. B., Chitwood, D. D., Smith, P. C., & McBride, D. C. 1990a. Intravenous drug abuse and HIV infection in Miami. *Medical Anthropology Quarterly 4(1):* 56–71.

Page, J. B., Smith, P. C., & Kane, N. 1990b. Venous envy: The importance of having functional veins. *Journal of Drug Issues 20(2):* 287–304.

Page, J. B., Smith, P. C., & Kane, N. 1990c. Shooting galleries, their proprietors, and implications for prevention of AIDS. *Drugs and Society, 5* (1/2): 69–85.

Polsky, N. 1967. Research method, mortality, and criminology. In: N. Polsky, *Hustlers, Beats, and Others.* New York: Anchor, pp. 109–143.

Ridder, L. 1981. Qualitative research and quasi-experimental frameworks. In: M. Brewer & B. Collins, eds., *Scientific Inquiry and the Social Sciences.* San Francisco, CA: Jossey Bass.

Sandstrom, K. L. 1990. Confronting deadly disease: The drama of identity construction among gay men with AIDS. *Journal of Contemporary Ethnography 19:* 271–294.

Spradley, J. 1980. *Participant Observation.* New York: Holt, Rinehart, and Winston.

Stall, R., Heurtin-Roberts, S., McCusick, L., Hoff, C., Mouton, J., & Lang, S. 1990. Sexual risk for HIV infection among bar patrons in San Francisco. *Medical Anthropology Quarterly 4(1):* 115–128.

Stimson, G. 1989. Syringe-exchange programmes for injection drug users. *AIDS 3:* 253–260.

Strauss, A. 1987. *Qualitative Analyses for Social Scientists.* New York: Cambridge University Press.

Strauss, A., & Corbin, J. 1990. *Basics of Qualitative Research: Grounded Theory Procedures and Techniques.* London: Sage.

Tesch, R. 1989. *Qualitative Research: Analyses Types and Software Tools.* Philadelphia, PA: Taylor and Francis.

Tesch, R. 1991. Introduction to the special issue, computers and qualitative data II. *Qualitative Sociology 14:* 225–243.

Walters, J. 1980. What is ethnography? In: C. Akins and G. Beschner, eds., *Ethnography: A Research Tool for Policy Makers in the Drug and Alcohol Fields.* Rockville, MD: National Institute on Drug Abuse, pp. 15–20.

Watters, S. K. 1989. Observations on the importance of social context in HIV transmission among intravenous drug users. *Journal of Drug Issues 19:* 9–26.

Wilkelstein, W., Samuel, M., Padian, N. S., Wiley, J. A., Lang, W., Anderson, W. E., & Levy, J. A. 1987. The San Francisco mens' health study: III. Reduction in human immunodeficiency virus transmission among homosexual/bisexual men, 1982–1986. *American Journal of Public Health 77:* 685–689.

Williams, T., Dunlap, E., Johnson, B. D., & Hamid, A. 1992. Personal safety in dangerous places. *Journal of Contemporary Ethnography 21(3):* 343–374.

Worth, D. 1989. Sexual decision making and AIDS: Why condom promotion among vulnerable women is likely to fail. *Studies of Family Planning 20(6):* 297–307.

Worth, D. 1990a. Minority women and AIDS: Culture, race and gender. In: D. Feldman, ed., *Culture and AIDS.* New York: Praeger, pp. 111–135.

Worth, D. 1990b. Women at high risk of HIV infection: Behavioral, prevention and intervention aspects. In: D. Ostrow, ed., *Behavioral Aspects of AIDS and other STD's.* New York: Plenum Press, pp. 101–119.

Designing an Intervention Study

Jose Szapocznik and Willo Pequegnat

Traditionally, an intervention has been construed as a set of activities on the part of an "intervenor" to bring about changes in the behavior of target individuals or groups. There are three major paradigms for behavior change: (1) mechanistic (e.g., Skinnerian models); (2) organismic (e.g., Piagetian, Freudian models); and (3) contextual (e.g., family systems, cultural models). With the recent advent of contextualism, theories of behavior change have been expanded to include cultural factors that influence behavior. Social learning theory, which has been widely used in HIV prevention research, has been subsumed under a contextual paradigm.

This chapter provides guidance on the steps in designing an HIV-related intervention research study. In addition to discussing the complexities involved at each step, important methodological issues, discussed in more detail in other chapters in this book, are also raised (see Table 1).

Statement of the Problem

Our interest in designing an intervention does not exist in a vacuum, but is mobilized when we identify a problem that needs to be addressed. A problem can range from behaviors that place white gay men at risk for HIV transmission to issues of psychological and family adjustment confronted by minority pregnant women who are HIV positive.

In developing the intervention, it is essential to develop a descriptive statement of the problem. The statement of the problem is closely linked to your theoretical framework, because the way that a problem is conceptualized is intimately related to the lens (theory) through which it is viewed, and it is beneficial to consider several approaches before making a final selection. For example, you may decide that the nature of the problem with white gay men who engage in HIV high-risk behavior is in their attitudes (an interpersonal cognitive lens); or, alternatively, the problem may be social norms in which these men are embedded (a contextual lens). Similarly, in understanding the problem of HIV-positive minority pregnant adolescents, we may be primarily concerned with the behavior of the youth herself, or, alternatively, we

**Table 1. Designing
an Intervention**

Statement of the problem
Study population
Points of intervention
Literature search
Theoretical framework
Pre-application work
Unit of intervention
Types of variables
    independent variables
    dependent variables
    mediating and moderating variables
Standardizing the intervention
    dosage
    nature of sessions
    intervenors
    manual
Internal and external validity
    control group
    maturation
    history
    non-specific effects
    differential mortality
Usefulness of intervention studies
Consensus on preventive interventions

may be concerned with the contextual circumstances that discourage this young woman from developing a sense of empowerment and direction about her own life.

Study Population

A problem is usually defined in relationship to a population. In fact, for those of us in applied work, typically we begin working with a population, and then discover specific problems. We then become interested in conducting an intervention (the solution to the problem) and in testing its effectiveness (intervention research).

If you have read any of the federal Program Announcements or Requests for Applications recently, you know that the subject variable of ethnicity/race and gender must be addressed in research applications submitted for federal funding. It is challenging to address these issues adequately in a research design because different ethnic/race and gender groups have specific characteristics and needs. It may be necessary to make important adjustments to psychosocial interventions in order to ensure that they are appropriate across a range of ethnic/racial and gender groups. The intervention may be closely tied to cultural or gender characteristics. For example, an intervention aimed at a college-educated population may build on their cognitive orientation, whereas an intervention targeting recent immigrant Hispanic grandmothers may build on their interpersonal orientation.

Points of Intervention

In considering the nature of the problem, it is also important to decide at what point in its development you want to intervene. Would you like to intervene to avoid HIV transmission (primary prevention)? Would you want to intervene early in the process of HIV infection to enhance adjustment, improve quality of life, and delay progression (secondary prevention)? Or would you like to intervene in the treatment and rehabilitation of symptomatic individuals, such as in developing care for individuals affected with AIDS dementia (tertiary intervention)? Table 2 provides a brief definition of each of the three types of prevention/intervention strategies.

Literature Search

Once you have developed your own ideas about the problem, your next step is to learn about the knowledge base that exists in the research literature. Even if you do not agree with the existing scientific base, your scientific inquiry should be based on the best available scientific data. The literature review is not a one-time search but an ongoing process that begins as soon as the problem is defined and continues each time a new aspect of the problem emerges during the study.

Topics that are relevant to designing your intervention include the target population and its culture, the nature of the problem, theoretical or conceptual frameworks that could be invoked to develop solutions to the problem, and methods to measure outcomes due to the intervention.

Although your concerns may be specifically with AIDS, useful information on potential efficacious interventions with other chronic diseases (e.g., cancer or diabetes mellitus) or models of behavior change that have been successful in the past can be useful. Models range from the frequently used brief, cognitively oriented interventions in HIV prevention to clinical interventions based on psychodynamic, family systems, or behavior theory to community-wide interventions (e.g., smoking cessation, cancer, and substance abuse prevention).

Table 2. Definitions of Prevention

Primary Prevention Focuses on reducing the occurrence of known or suspected causative factors of mental or physical illness.

Secondary Prevention Focuses on efforts at early detection and treatment through examination, testing, and adherence to a treatment regimen

Tertiary Prevention Focuses on rehabilitation from the effects of the mental or physical health problem

While it is important to review the literature in order to design your study, it is also important to demonstrate to the review committee that you have mastered the relevant literature. The reviewer needs to know not only the reasons that you chose a particular approach but also why you ruled out other alternatives. For example, you may discuss several potential theoretical frameworks that could be used to explain a particular phenomenon, and then explain why you chose one of these over the others.

Theoretical Framework

A theory is a way of explaining the nature of the problem and the assumptions that you make about the nature of the problem, which suggests interventions to address the problem.[1] In fact, the theoretical framework becomes the organizing force for a research study. Once selected, it has implications for how the problem is framed (lens) and what the solution might be (intervention), as well as for the kinds of variables to be included in the study (e.g., independent, dependent, mediating, and moderating variables).

In this section, we would like to explore briefly the role of theory in selecting an intervention. Take the example of designing a preventive intervention for Hispanic adolescent gang members in the age group of 12 to 15. Many HIV-preventive intervention programs are based on social learning theory that makes assumptions about behavior change linked to certain variables, including cognitions, self-efficacy, and perceived social norms. Hence, if we choose this theoretical framework, we would design an intervention that targets appropriate variables for this adolescent population.

In order to reduce high-risk behaviors in risk-seeking adolescents with a sense of omnipotence, another theoretical framework might suggest targeting their sense of self-worth. An intervention encouraging a parent to communicate a nonambiguous message of "I love you" might be instrumental in encouraging adolescents to be receptive to other messages about caring for her or his health.

Other theoretical approaches, such as those based on family systems theory, might suggest that the risk-seeking/acting-out behavior in some adolescents is a symptom of family interactional patterns. Thus, an intervention might be designed to promote family communication that reduces family stress and enhances the family's ability to set behavioral limits. Such interventions might include creating clear and firm rules and consequences for acting-out behaviors, improving communication and negotiation skills, increasing positive affect, enhancing parental leadership, decreasing outside family stressors, and increasing outside family support systems.

While the previous three examples were based on psychosocial theories, we might seek a biological explanation for the problem. We might suggest that risk-seeking youths suffer from "understimulation," and their behavior can best be explained as a need to regulate a biological process that seeks a certain level of arousal. Other potential biological theories, such as notions of serotonergic system dysfunction, are also possible. Clearly, either one of these biological assumptions would lead to different interventions.

Our understanding of the nature of a problem is critical in selecting the theoretical framework to explain the problem and organize our intervention. An assumption that information is needed to change behavior or that changes in social norms will induce behavior change will lead to dramatically different choices for a theoretical model than those based on power relationships, multisystem problems, or biological assumptions.

---

[1] Editors' note: See "Developing a Theoretical Framework and Rationale for a Research Proposal" by Herek, this volume.

Pre-Application Work

There are three areas in which pre-application pilot work may be needed: (1) to familiarize yourself with the target population; (2) to assess the feasibility of your protocol; and (3) to establish potential efficacy for the proposed intervention.

Target Population

In designing interventions, there are two common mistakes committed by new investigators. One is the investigator who knows a theoretical or intervention approach and thinks it would be interesting to apply it to a new problem. The other is the investigator who comes from the same population as the target group and understands what makes this population "tick," but does not have sufficient objectivity to describe the population. Both of these investigators would benefit from conducting a pilot study. If they are right, then they can marshall data to convince the review committee. If they are wrong, they will have been spared the time of investing in a fruitless effort.

In your pre-application work, you may want to conduct small studies to learn more about the population. These studies may range from survey to clinical, from quantitative to qualitative, depending on the nature of the information you want to pursue. If you already know about the population because you come from the same group, you still need to develop a database on the population so that you can support your observations or conjectures. On the other hand, if you do not know the population, then you need to become familiar with your chosen group of interest and demonstrate this in your application. The strategy that you use in obtaining data will depend on the kind of information that you are seeking. For example, if you want to know what kinds of behaviors place individuals in a specific group at risk for HIV transmission, you might collect epidemiologic-type data on HIV risk behaviors for that group.

While a survey may tell you what behavior to target, it does not tell you how to design your intervention. For example, if you find that gay teenagers engage in unprotected anal intercourse because they think that most teenagers are uninfected, you may decide to develop an intervention that presents information to gay teenagers on the true risks. Such an intervention may work with some teenagers and not with others, because, while information is necessary, it often is not sufficient. After all, it is not uncommon to find teenagers who are well-informed about the risks of cigarette smoking, crack cocaine, carrying weapons, gang membership, speeding when driving, or drinking and driving who are still engaging in these high-risk behaviors. Hence, a deeper understanding of life-span development and a more profound understanding of clinical issues involving high-risk behavior may be helpful. Knowledge of these phenomena may be better developed with more in-depth clinical and qualitative interviews with representative members from the target population, rather than through survey studies.

Feasibility of Protocol

Clearly, the purpose of the intervention study is to determine whether the investigator's idea for an intervention will work. But the investigator needs to convince a group of scientists reviewing the application that the intervention is scientifically credible and feasible. One of the paradoxes in submitting a grant application is that, if you propose a study that has been conducted before (called a replication), the scientists reviewing your proposal may think it is not original, and thus you will have to convince them of the importance of a replication. On the other hand, if you are proposing an untested intervention or one that has not been used with your target population, you will have to convince them that the intervention

Table 3. Intervention Strategies for Changing High-Risk Behavior

Modality	Clinical	Institutional	Community
Target	Individual	Schools, businesses, prisons	Cities, regions, TV markets
Method	One-on-one, family, or group therapy	Group discussions, brochures	TV and radio magazine and newspapers, public speakers

can be implemented and may be effective. In the latter case, you will need to conduct a pilot study in order to demonstrate on a small scale that the larger study has the potential for success. However, another very valuable purpose of the pilot study is to provide you with information that will help you refine both your intervention and other aspects of the procedures involved in conducting a rigorous intervention study.

Potential Efficacy

Finally, a pilot study can provide you with information on the scale of the impact or "effect size" that can be expected for an intervention with a specific sample. The effect size is important because it is needed to calculate the number of subjects that you will need in the intervention to achieve sufficient power to test your hypotheses.[2]

Unit of Intervention

In designing an intervention, we must decide whether we will intervene at the level of individuals, groups, small natural social networks, or even entire communities. Table 3 provides a taxonomy of intervention strategies. The unit of intervention is an important decision which should be made on substantive or theoretical grounds, that is, what will work best based on our knowledge of the problem and the population.

Another reason to choose a particular unit of intervention is based on cost-benefit analysis. We may believe that an individual approach will be more likely to help each individual, but if there are limited resources and a group approach can help a substantial proportion of the participants, this may be the more cost-effective method. This rationale comes from the field of public health, which is concerned with creating the greatest benefit for the largest number of persons, even though everyone may not be helped equally or maximally.

The selection of a unit of intervention may have implications for data analyses. This is a relatively complex statistical/methodological issue. In brief, however, the rule is that if individuals are randomly assigned to various interventions, then individuals are the unit of analysis. If, on the other hand, you randomly assign communities to the intervention or non-intervention, then your unit for data analysis becomes the entire community. In order to attain sufficient statistical power to enable you to test your hypotheses formally, you would need a large number of communities.[3]

[2] Editors' note: See "How Do You Formulate a Testable Exciting Hypothesis?" by Dawes, this volume.
[3] Editors' note: See "Developing the Data Analytic Plan" by Taylor, this volume.

Types of Variables

Independent Variables

There are several types of variables that are included in research studies. Some of these, such as independent and dependent variables, are basic to all studies. Other variables, such as mediating and moderating variables, may not be used in all studies. All four types of variables, however, are closely linked, if not dictated, by the theoretical framework selected.

Intervention outcome studies are usually intended to investigate if the intervention causes an effect. The variable associated with the effect is referred to as the independent variable; the effect is assessed by changes in the dependent variable. Selecting the specific constructs for both of these kinds of variables is guided by the theoretical framework.

There are a broad range of potential independent or predictor variables. The most common independent variable in an intervention study is the manipulated intervention/control condition. However, many other predictor variables are included in intervention studies. Some of these include characteristics of the session leader (e.g., peer versus authority figure), dosage (e.g., four versus eight sessions), form of administration (e.g., massed [all at once] versus spaced [one session per week]), pre-intervention conditions, and subject characteristics.

The most common independent variable used in an intervention study is the intervention condition itself. That is, usually we hypothesize that the intervention will have an expected effect. In this case, the condition in which the intervention was applied is our experimental condition, while the condition in which the intervention was not applied is our control condition. The independent variable in this case is "condition."

The aim of most intervention studies is to establish that there is a specific factor that is accounting for the effect. This is both an issue of definition of the independent variable as well as an issue of internal validity, described in a subsequent section. That is, if an intervention works, we want to know what made it work so that it is replicable. Was it the warmth and attention of a caring professional that caused the effect, or was it something about the specific techniques that were employed? In research terms, we would refer to these contributions to an effect as nonspecific (e.g., warmth, attention) versus specific (e.g., the four educational sessions provided).

Subject variables, individual difference variables, are sufficiently important to deserve careful consideration. It is very common in intervention research to ask the question: "If it works, with whom does it work, and under what conditions?" According to our theoretical framework, we may be able to make predictions about certain kinds of subjects that are most likely to benefit from the intervention. For example, it may be very different to encourage safer sex with individuals who are in a power position in a relationship than with those who are disempowered. When we believe that some subjects may benefit more than others, we might choose to limit the intervention to those we think will benefit. However, there are advantages to including subjects that we believe may or may not benefit in order to establish the specificity of an intervention (i.e., the fact that it works with some persons with specific characteristics and not with others).[4]

Dependent Variables

The theoretical model should also guide the selection of dependent variables in order to assess those factors that we intend to impact as a result of our intervention. In the case of HIV, the most frequently

[4] Editors' note: See "How Do You Formulate a Testable Exciting Hypothesis?" by Dawes, this volume.

assessed dependent variables are HIV-related high-risk behaviors, adjustment to learning about one's serostatus, and immunological variations and/or disease progression. Of course, the dependent variable is closely tied to the nature of the problem. When the problem is high-risk sexual behavior, then it is this behavior that we wish to change, and thus it becomes our dependent variable. However, if we are conducting an intervention to improve psychological adjustment, then measures of psychological adjustment are our dependent variable. Other dependent variables of interest in HIV could include family adjustment to learning that one of its members is HIV positive, community reactions to persons with HIV/AIDS, and parenting of HIV antibody-positive infants.

Mediating and Moderating Variables

Mediating and moderating variables can also be important in designing intervention studies. A mediating variable is one that we believe may be a pathway to the desired outcome; for example, we may hypothesize that a change in social norms will lead to behavior change. Our intervention will target changing social norms, and our ultimate dependent variable will be changes in high-risk behaviors. However, it would be useful to measure the mediating variable, social norms, to determine the extent to which changes in social norms, in fact, accounted for the variance found in our ultimate outcome, changes in high-risk behaviors. In this fashion, we are able to test our basic assumptions or theory as well.

Moderating variables tend to interact in some fashion to alter the relationship between an independent and a dependent variable. One example of the importance of moderating variables is found in HIV-related psychoneuroimmunological studies. In these studies, there has been an interest in determining the condition under which stress (independent variable) is likely to result in distress and decreased immunological functioning (dependent variables). However, some investigators have identified two variables, coping style and social support, that may moderate the effects of stress on measures of distress and immunological functioning. Hence, the impact of stress on the predicted outcomes depends on how a subject copes with the stress and the extent of the subject's social support system. In designing an intervention study around stress, understanding the moderating variables is crucial. In fact, it may be that our primary intervention would be targeted not at the independent factor (stress) but, rather, at the variables that moderate it (coping and social support).

Standardizing the Intervention

There are many difficult and complex issues involved in designing an intervention research study. One of the most complex issues is the standardization of the intervention. The intervention should be defined so that its basic parameters are thoroughly described. This description should be sufficiently well detailed so that other professionals with your training are able to implement the intervention at their sites.

The problem with the level of specificity provided by most new investigators reflects the difficulty in specifying exactly what the intervention entails. When writing the description, investigators often fail to include factors that are essential components in implementing the intervention.

In the following sections some important issues in achieving standardization are discussed: intensity of the intervention, nature of sessions, intervenors, the manual, and quality assurance.

Intensity of Intervention

Interventions are defined in a number of ways. One way that we design interventions is in terms of the form, frequency, and intensity of administration of the intervention (i.e., dosage). In selecting a particular dosage, there should be a rationale that explains why you believe it is optimum. You may decide to conduct only one session because you cannot retain your subjects over multiple sessions or because you want to begin with the most parsimonious intervention. You may plan six sessions because that is the number that you have found to be effective with your population in preventing other STDs. In either case, the question of the minimum number of sessions that will be sufficiently intense to have the desired effect must be addressed.

The question of dosage is particularly complex in addressing certain kinds of problems. Some interventions lend themselves to crisp definitions, such as applying social learning theory–based interventions to educate white gay men in an intervention to reduce high-risk sexual behavior. An initial intervention involving four group intervention sessions delivered at regular intervals of approximately a week apart has been suggested as an adequate dosage.

On the other hand, when working with a chronic condition such as HIV infection, specifying the dosage for an intervention to address the evolving mental health needs of a population presents special challenges of standardization across all subjects in the intervention condition. In these cases, it is still necessary to present a replicable intervention, but the replicability may be a decision tree based on the emerging needs of the individual. Hence, it is not the dosage that is standardized across subjects, but the procedure by which decisions about how to administer certain aspects and dosages of the intervention are made. This is not unlike the problems that are confronted in medical trials with complex, multiproblem, and chronic conditions in which dosage needs to be titrated to maximize clinical effects and minimize undesirable side effects.

Nature of the Sessions

Whatever the nature of your intervention, two aspects must be specified to ensure that the intervention is replicable and acceptable for use in a research: content and process. Content refers to the actual topics of discussion, whereas process refers to the activities, interactions, and method of delivery.

In the specification of the nature of sessions, the investigator lays out the curriculum and behavioral expectations for each session. However, content does not explain all that transpires in any intervention and that may account for impact. Take, for example, teaching classes in schools. The identical textbook and teacher's manual can be used by teachers throughout an entire school system. Yet, some teachers will be more successful than others. Clearly, content describes what is taught, but it does not address the way that teachers create hope, expectation, enthusiasm, and eagerness to learn. And it reveals little about the ability of the teacher to use different strategies to reach children who are motivated by different needs. Thus, to capture what happens in an intervention, it is important to describe the process as well as the content, paying attention to those behaviors on the part of the intervenor that are crucial to the success of the intervention. Explaining all of these aspects should be explicit, because it will be used to train the intervenors, conduct the sessions, and monitor adherence to the parameters of intervention.

We have been assuming that the interventions are designed so that they can be applied in a modular format that we call "sessions." The nature of the intervention may be difficult to define in community-wide interventions where the modules are not of sessions, but of complex activities, such as the steps in an HIV prevention media campaign. If we are rigorous in preparing the manual, we need to specify how we initiate collaboration with the media, which represents a complex set of behaviors from describing abstract concepts in a prevention campaign to engaging the power structure and marketing a concept to the media and other community decision-makers.

As mentioned earlier, a crucial aspect of constructing an intervention that can be used for research is to ensure its replicability. The factors that facilitate the replicability of an intervention are debatable. Clearly, if we are teaching a child the multiplication tables, we can clearly specify the content. There are also intangible concepts that have to be described as part of an intervention, which are difficult to explain in concrete terms. For example, determining what a child's needs are and how to meet them are crucial to ensuring that the child will learn multiplication tables, but it involves relatively abstract behaviors on the part of the intervenor.

Intervenors

Persons involved in conducting an intervention are crucial to its success. Careful consideration needs to be given to their professional expertise, level of training, interpersonal skills, and personal qualities.

The appropriate characteristics for intervenors may vary widely depending on the nature of the intervention and its theoretical underpinnings. For example, in a community-wide intervention using mass media to target condom use, the "intervenors" are a team of individuals whose expertise ranges from media to behavior change to marketing to public relations and community organization. In this instance, it would be difficult to train an individual to do an adequate job if that person does not already possess many of the prerequisite skills and contacts. On the other hand, in an intervention study using social learning theory with white gay men, intervenors are likely to be members of the target population who administer a relatively simple psychoeducational program. Finally, in a mental health intervention with inner-city, African-American HIV-positive pregnant women, the intervenors need to have basic training in systems theory and considerable experience in work with African-American women and their families. In these latter two cases, it may be possible to train persons with good interpersonal skills to conduct the standardized intervention in a relatively brief time.

Possessing the basic skills for delivering an intervention is not always sufficient; the intervenor must also be able to adhere to implementing the intervention in a standardized way. This includes doing both what is minimally required as the basic, specific ingredients of the intervention as well as not doing things that are not permitted by the intervention model. Deviations in either of these directions are threats to the internal validity of a study and reduce its replicability.

In our experience, many intervenors with applied experience are initially eager to participate in a research study. However, when they are confronted with the restrictions and demands of the actual study, they find themselves in conflict with their intuitive style of conducting groups, rather than following a set of protocol guidelines. Hence, it is important to select intervenors who are fully aware of the protocol guidelines, understand its demands and constraints, and are committed to implementing it as specified. This is possible if the intervenor understands that documenting the validity of an approach will ultimately help more people than can be touched directly.

Manual

The *sine qua non* of intervention research is the manual accompanying the intervention, which specifies the critical aspects of the intervention. Many manuals resemble an agenda. This is inadequate because a manual needs to provide guidelines and strategies for conducting the intervention. It needs to specify what can be done, what must be done, and what should not be done. It also needs to discuss issues of content and process. To repeat, a manual should have the necessary information to permit intervenors of similar backgrounds to implement essentially the same intervention by strictly following the manual guidelines.

Quality Assurance

The first four issues discussed under achieving standardization address quality control, which sets out the guidelines or rules for conducting the intervention. Quality assurance is the procedures set in place to ensure that the guidelines are followed across intervenors and at the various sites where the intervention is conducted.

Internal and External Validity

In this section it is our intention to provide an overview of the complexity of conducting intervention research on difficult problems. There is an old adage in research that internal and external validity are inversely related. The more closely you develop a study that reflects the external reality (external validity), the more difficult it will be to have a rigorous design (internal validity), and vice versa. It is impossible to give simple formulas for how to strike the best balance. This is a decision that each investigator must make based on the desire to conduct a study that is generalizable versus one that is rigorous.

Control Group

The purpose of a control condition is to permit you to rule out alternative explanations of your findings. There are different kinds of control conditions (e.g., no intervention, wait-list, placebo, alternative intervention, etc.), and there has been considerable debate about the desirability of different types for different research purposes. There are no easy answers, and the selection of a control condition will depend on the nature of the problem, the population, and the plausible alternative explanations.

In this section we highlight the difficulties inherent in maintaining the purity of control conditions. This is particularly important when control conditions provide minimal or no intervention. In this case, contamination of the control condition with intervention effects can be particularly harmful because the results might suggest that a no-intervention control condition was effective.

An example from AIDS research of contamination of a structural change that had an impact on both the experimental and control group may be illustrative, although the structural change was not controlled by the investigators.

You may be familiar with the NIDA AIDS Demonstration Projects. In one part of the project, injection drug users (IDUs) are assigned randomly to either the control condition, where they receive a one-time brief educational intervention, or an enhanced condition, where, in addition to the brief session, they receive three additional sessions of advanced education. The IDUs living in some cities tend to frequent shooting galleries. For this example, let us say that the owner of one of the shooting galleries is assigned to the enhanced intervention, and the enhanced intervention is in fact effective. The owner of the shooting gallery therefore changes the rules so that everybody who shoots there has to clean their needles.

Then we have a second person who was assigned to the control condition, which is not effective. This man, however, is a customer of the shooting gallery owned by the man who received the enhanced condition. Although this second man is in the control group, he goes to a shooting gallery that is being ruled by someone in the enhanced group, which means that the experimental intervention is diffusing to the control condition. Thus, some control people do better than expected because they are impacted by an experimental structural change. This is a problem in maintaining the purity of the control condition. We could have solved it by randomly assigning subjects by networks, rather than as individuals, in order to limit contamination across treatment conditions. However, it might not have been possible to assign randomly by network because we may not have been able to recruit a sufficient number of networks to achieve sufficient analytic power.

Another example of the way that control conditions become contaminated is based on an intervention study to test the effect of different types of social support interventions on immunological functioning. Persons infected with HIV would be randomly assigned to a condition where they would receive enhanced social support and to a control condition where they would not. However, the people in the control group may feel needy, and there is no way of keeping them from seeking social support.

An alternative would be to exclude needy people based on some measure of "neediness." We would only recruit subjects who are not too needy in both conditions; if they were in the no-treatment group, they would presumably be able to cope on their own well enough to stay in the program without seeking enhanced social support. But if we do that, we may have a selection bias problem because we have enrolled a sample of only "moderately needy people." The question can be raised that our intervention may not be effective with very high or very low levels of "neediness." This is another example where scientific rigor may be at odds with generalizability of the results.

Maturation

There are several other potential threats that must be considered in designing interventions in AIDS research. If you are working with HIV infection, one of the threats to the validity of an intervention study is maturation, because people who are infected with HIV may be improving in response to pharmacologic therapy or deteriorating in the course of their illness. If you conduct an intervention and do not have a control group, your aggregate finding may be that everybody is more or less the same a year later. You might then conclude that your intervention had no impact, but, if you had a control group, you might find that the control group actually deteriorated more rapidly and your intervention was effective in slowing or preventing deterioration. This was the case with AZT studies, where, without the control group, the early conclusion might have been that this anti-retroviral drug was of little or no benefit.

History

History is another consideration in designing studies, and a difficult issue to control if you are conducting community intervention studies. A good example of this is the intervention efforts in San Francisco within the gay community. The belief is that gay people changed their behaviors due to the massive educational campaign. There are other ways of explaining what happened in San Francisco, however. For example, if each gay man in San Francisco knows between 10 and 50 people who have died of AIDS, then perhaps the historical set of events—exposure to a disaster where so many friends died—may have brought about the change in sexual behavior (rather than the educational intervention). Thus, historical threats to intervention studies are incredibly important yet difficult to control in large community studies.

Nonspecific Effects

Most research studies are designed to demonstrate that a specific effect or active ingredient is necessary to bring about a desired outcome. We have already discussed the distinction between specific and nonspecific effects above.

There is an area of investigation in HIV, particularly related to the field of psychoneuroimmunology, that departs radically from the usual practice in intervention research. In these studies, the nonspecific effects, such as placebo, expectancy, and attention, are not considered nuisances to be controlled by attention/placebo control conditions. Rather, in psychoneuroimmunology these are considered important factors with potential for generating desired outcomes, such as improved immune function and health. In this case, it is crucial for the investigator to distinguish between the kinds of research designs in which it is desirable to control for the traditional nonspecific effects and those in which these effects are deemed worthy of pursuit as powerful predictor or intervening variables.

Differential Mortality

The last threat to internal validity we would like to discuss in this section is differential mortality. When you read the literature on interventions, data are often not provided on the number of people who did not finish in each condition unless "an intention to treat" strategy is adopted. Instead, results are reported only for those people who completed the different intervention or control conditions. Persons may have dropped out for reasons that were independent of the intervention (e.g., to take care of a sick friend, etc.). On the other hand, attrition may have occurred that biased the results. For example, persons may have been sicker and/or could not handle the rigors of the intervention or may have died and are no longer available at the time of post-testing. In the latter case, the apparent success of the intervention may be due to the stamina and better health of the persons who completed the study and the fact that those who could not tolerate the intervention dropped out.

An example of misleading results that can occur when there is differential attrition is based on epidemiologic studies of adolescent drug use. The issue of differential mortality has been discussed in studies that have estimated drug abuse rates among high school seniors. The data indicate that, among high school seniors surveyed, Hispanics and non-Hispanic whites have about the same rate of drug use. But what the data do not say is that about 10 percent of the white students dropped out of school, while about 40 percent of the Hispanic students dropped out. We know that there is a higher rate of drug abuse among students who drop out of school. If your study only recruited adolescents who were in school, both ethnic groups would appear to be similar on drug use patterns, but if you include adolescents who dropped out of school, then you might conclude that Hispanic youth have higher drug use rates. The issue of how you handle differential mortality is important in the credibility of your results.

One way of addressing the differential mortality problem in your grant proposal is to be candid. For example, if you suspect that it is impossible to have a representative sample on a longitudinal basis, then the only methodologically sound study may be cross-sectional. Another option is to propose pursuing some of your dropouts, but this depends on how intrusive you want to be, presuming that they are alive. Intrusive follow-up of dropouts raises ethical concerns, some of which can be addressed by the nature of the contract you establish with your subjects about permission to pursue them for follow ups.

Consensus on Preventative Interventions

The Office on AIDS, National Institute of Mental Health, sponsors an annual meeting of AIDS prevention researchers involved in the development and evaluation of behavioral strategies to prevent the further spread of HIV. The consensus is that: (1) AIDS prevention programs are more successful if they are integrated into ongoing systems of care (e.g., STD clinic, family medicine clinics, etc.); (2) prevention strategies should be tailored to the specific population, should involve participation by the community, and should be led by persons with whom the participants can identify; and (3) in the hierarchy of concerns of persons at risk for HIV infection, housing, crime, and unemployment may rank higher than HIV risk and may need to be addressed prior to implementing HIV prevention programs. Some of these guidelines for designing interventions are presented in Table 4.

To highlight the complexity between integrating work in the real world with theoretical and empirical research, it is worth noting that the investigators provide a set of recommendations that may reflect the conflict between research and practice. For example, research in HIV prevention has tended to be based on social learning theory, yet practice suggests that this cognitively oriented theoretical model may not adequately address the hierarchy of real life concerns of inner city minority populations, which confront multiple contextual problems. Other models for appropriate interventions will need to be explored in the second decade of AIDS research.

Table 4. Designing Appropriate Intervention Programs[a]

Community models using social marketing techniques and diffusion of innovation theory have also been successful.

Researchers who plan to intervene in an institution (e.g., schools) should have a history of working within that system.

For hard-to-reach individuals at high risk, programs need to go where they are, not expect people to come to prevention programs.

Prevention programs should be integrated into ongoing systems of care (e.g., STD clinics, family medicine clinics, etc.).

Advocacy to meet the basic needs of persons (e.g., housing, food, medical care, etc.) must be done at the same time as prevention.

Community people must participate in the design of the intervention program in order to tailor it to the specific needs of the local community.

Different people respond to different levels of interventions; some people respond to low intensity, while others require one-on-one or small group interventions.

Timing is important in successful interventions; it is easier to change high-risk sexual behaviors at the beginning of a new relationship than in an ongoing one.

Women at high risk may need nonthreatening community settings that also address physical and sexual abuse issues in the context of HIV prevention.

Problem behaviors are often found in clusters with adolescent populations (e.g., smoking, alcohol, drugs, teen pregnancy).

For preadolescents, it is important to change determinants of high-risk behavior.

In order to prevent relapse to high-risk behaviors, the social environment of the person may need to be changed.

Initiate relapse prevention strategies should be built into the initial intervention.

[a] Editors' note: This is a summary based on a meeting of 21 NIMH Principal Investigators on Prevention, April 8–10, 1991.

Usefulness of Intervention Studies

There has been considerable debate about the lack of overlap between what is done in actual mental health practice and what is the subject of research. In the psychotherapy research field, for example, there has been considerable concern that the kinds of mental health interventions that are most prevalent in the country are not well represented in mental health research. Most research studies, in fact, use modular interventions, in which content is construed as more important than process and that can be administered to large numbers of subjects in relatively few sessions.

There are two streams of thought about the discrepancy between actual mental health care and research conducted on mental health interventions. One stream suggests that, if we can demonstrate that "containerized" interventions work, they are likely to be adapted by the field. Another stream of thought, however, is concerned about the lack of willingness of researchers to conduct mental health intervention research that reflects the wisdom of the clinical field and that evaluates existing mental health intervention models.

There are many challenges presented by both of these approaches. Moreover, it is challenging to attempt to "containerize" mental health interventions that resemble clinical practice and are likely to incorporate theoretical and clinical concepts and processes that require a considerable level of abstraction.

Conclusions

In this brief chapter, we have attempted to raise some of the complex issues involved in conducting intervention research in general as well as specifically in AIDS. The issues are many, and the complexity of this area is challenging.

Our intent is to encourage new researchers to become involved in this difficult field. We have attempted to be candid about the enormous obstacles in attempting to design relevant intervention studies. We have made the point several times throughout the chapter that our own bias is to encourage relevant research, and yet we recognize that to the extent that research is designed to reflect reality, it may lose some rigor and may compromise the validity of the findings. Hence, we warn the prospective investigator that this is a field in which a delicate balance between rigor and relevance must be maintained. It is our professional challenge to design the most rigorous and relevant studies that we can, while not despairing when we are forced to give up relevance for rigor in order to move the scientific field forward. Remember that you will not be able to investigate all the important variables in one study. Rather, science is built on one small finding at a time. Thus, design your studies to address a specific hypothesis, and do not try to address every issue in a single study.

13

Instrumentation
Off the Shelf or on Your Own

Robert Remien

Measurement and instrumentation are often viewed as minor considerations in the broader picture of research design, but they can be crucial to your project's potential success. The quality of your research will depend on the quality of the data you collect, which, in turn, will depend on the psychometric properties of the measures you use. Many prospective applicants have struggled with issues concerning measurement and instrumentation. You may have confronted problems as you searched for available measures and tried to decide which ones were appropriate for your population. You may also have concluded that none of them were appropriate or could be adapted for your study and decided to design measures of your own.

The choice of measures used in your study will be influenced by many factors. This overview will focus on measurement issues most germane to applying for a research grant from NIMH, particularly in AIDS research.

To state the most obvious, the goals of your study will broadly determine what you choose to assess and how you choose to measure it. That is, your research questions will determine, for example, whether you will be making diagnostic assessments (e.g., mood disorders, personality disorders) or assessing severity of current psychiatric distress (e.g., depression or anxiety ratings); whether you will be measuring state or trait characteristics; whether you are concerned with change in behavior over time; or whether you will be looking at social supports, coping styles, stressful life events, or sex behaviors. These decisions are part of research design and will not be addressed in this chapter. Within your own content area, however, you will also need to make other choices about measurement, such as mode of assessment (i.e., self-report, structured interview, observer ratings). These types of decisions will depend on various factors above and beyond the goals of your study.

Measurement Review

In developing a research design, you first conduct a literature search; similarly, in measurement you should begin with a literature search for the appropriate instruments. However, because AIDS research is a fairly new field, you may not be able to rely on a well-established published literature. As a result, you may need to seek unpublished material or search the published literature in a related area of investigation. For example, to identify measures to assess people living with AIDS, it may be helpful to review measures that have been used in studies of cancer survivors.

Consulting with Other Investigators

An important step in the process is seeking consultation with other researchers. It is easier to ask for help in selecting measures than in designing the study because the questions you will ask of your consultant are more specific. You should seek consultation about measures after you know your research design and what you specifically want to measure. If possible, do not embark on developing your own measure because that can become a study in itself.

In seeking colleagues' recommendations, be clear about your constraints and be as specific as possible: "I need to measure severity of current depression in a way that includes few physical or vegetative symptoms. I will be assessing injection drug users (IDUs) who are predominantly Hispanic. I will have a B.A.-level person conducting the assessment, which must be completed within ½ hour." You are asking the consultants what they would recommend, given your goal, the constraints, and the context of your proposed research.

Budget for Measures

Funding, of course, is an issue in selecting measures. However, there is not only the cost of purchasing the instruments but also the costs of administering and scoring them. Inexperienced grant applicants often forget to include a budget for their measures, which usually must be purchased if they are copyrighted.

Staffing

Another important but often neglected issue is the level and quality of your staff. This should be an important part of your planning and your budgeting. The quality of your data depends not only on the measures you use but also on how well the data are collected. Therefore, the level of expertise and the quality of your interviewing or assessment staff are important.

Depending on your resources, the experience level of your staff (e.g., lay persons, B.A.s, M.A.s, Ph.D.s) will determine, in part, what measures you will choose. You will need to budget for appropriate level personnel depending on the objectives of your study. For example, if you want to assess the presence and/or severity of clinical depression or anxiety you would need experienced clinicians to administer something like a SCID (Structured Clinical Interview for DSM-III-R Diagnosis), a Hamilton Depression, or Anxiety Rating Scale. Alternatively, a trained lay person would be able to administer a DIS (Diagnostic Interview Schedule). If your resources are more limited, you may need to rely on the use of symptom rating scales that can be administered as self-reports, such as a Beck Depression or Anxiety Inventory or the BSI (Brief Symptom Inventory). Remember, different assessments require varying degrees of clinical judgment, ranging from none to high-level.

Training and Supervision

The training and supervision of staff is also an important and overlooked area in the process of selecting instruments. A principal investigator needs to be involved from the very beginning with the level of training and supervision of interviewing staff. If you are obtaining pilot data and are testing an instrument or a measure that will be adapted for the specific population under study, do not assume that your interviewing staff will identify discrepancies in data or the fact that an instrument's wording or language is inappropriate for your population.

Besides live supervision, the audiotaping of assessment interviews is recommended because it permits more direct contact with data collection. If you merely review the completed measures and scales or the coded data, but do not monitor how they are being administered and what is occurring in the interaction, you may be missing important information that will later assist you in interpreting your findings.

Discuss training and supervision in the proposal. Inform the reviewers, for example, "Our interviewers are going to be M.A.-level clinicians who will have been trained X number of hours. They will be supervised by a Ph.D. expert in psychiatric diagnosis."

Populations

There are considerations in selecting instruments for the populations you are studying. For example, measurements assess traditional variables—such as depression, anxiety, social supports, or stressful life events—but the wording or labels used may not be appropriate for your population. You might be measuring new kinds of behaviors, such as needle-sharing. You cannot, therefore, always rely on the availability of a standardized scale that has been used for years that can be applied successfully in your population. The wording of items may need to be modified, depending on the cultural or socioeconomic background or the sexual orientation of the people to whom you are administering it. If your population is gay men, for example, you may want to use the word "lover" instead of "spouse." Using items that are culturally specific helps to increase participants' motivation by making them feel that you recognize their unique identity.

The literacy level of your target population must be considered. Measures you choose and mode of administration must be appropriate to the reading level of your subjects.

It is very important to talk to other researchers and experts who have conducted investigations with the population you are studying and find out which measures have worked and which have not. If they have adapted a measure, get data from their study so you can compare your data.

Translation

If you need to have an instrument translated for your study population, you should be sensitive to the complexities of the process. It is not sufficient to have someone translate an instrument into another language; it must be tested by translation back into English. Also, you need to recognize regional variations in a language (e.g., Puerto Rican Spanish, Cuban Spanish, etc.).

You must also know the customs of the culture for which the translation is being made. Some concepts may not have an equivalent in another culture. An instrument in Spanish, for example, may need to be further adapted to ensure that it appropriately addresses the differing cultural as well as linguistic characteristics of the Hispanic populations being studied.

Confounds

While one must always consider potential confounds in measurement, a particular problem in the area of mental health assessment and HIV should be noted; it is the potential confounding of physical illness and psychiatric distress. Many "vegetative" symptoms are often included within some scales that measure depression or anxiety. How do you tease those symptoms out from what might be an effect of HIV infection on the individual? There are no quick-fix solutions or easy answers to this problem. You need to be aware of the problem, however, and choose measures accordingly, depending on your specific goals and interest. When measuring depression or anxiety, for example, you will probably have to decide whether to use a scale like the Hamilton Depression or Anxiety Scale, in which many items deal with potentially confounding physical symptoms (e.g., fatigue, weight loss, loss of appetite), or to rely on a more "cognitively" oriented scale such as the Beck Depression or Anxiety Inventory. If you decide to use a measure such as the Hamilton in a physically ill population, one suggestion is to allow for an "organic rule out," that is, to have an option where the rater can score for the presence of a symptom (e.g., weight loss) and then further decide whether they believe that the symptom is clearly and directly caused by the physical illness. The rater should indicate the organic factor (e.g., persistent diarrhea). This way in later analyses you can choose to look at the data, scored both ways, with and without counting these symptoms.

Using Standardized Measures versus Developing Your Own

If possible, beginning researchers should use standardized measures because psychometric properties have already been established and because there is a basis for believing that the instrument is measuring the construct of interest. In addition, your results can be compared to developed norms and also to results in other studies.

You should already have a basic understanding of the different types of validity and reliability of measurement and their importance in research. Sensitivity and specificity of measurement are also important psychometric properties you need to understand when doing some kinds of research. (See Freeman & Tyrer, 1989, for an excellent review of these issues.)

If necessary, explore modifying specific scales or see if someone else has modified them to make them more appropriate for your population. However, curb the urge to develop your own scales and questionnaires; reviewers may not be receptive to these novel instruments because they do not permit comparison to the general population. In general, do not undertake instrument development unless that is the focus of your proposal and the type of research you specifically want to do.

Instrument Modification or Adaptation

If you decide to adapt standardized measures to a particular population or setting, consult people who are doing research in the area. If possible, contact the person who developed the instrument you would like to use and say, "I want to use this instrument to measure social anxiety, but the population I plan to study is very different from the one on which this was normed. What do you think of these modifications?" Remember that if you make modifications, you will have to validate the instrument through a pilot study.

The more you modify or change a scale or instrument (e.g., altering the wording of the items or the mode of administration), the more you are moving away from the standardization upon which the instrument is based. Even if you take a scale that is typically a self-report and decide to administer it verbally (i.e., interviewer-assisted administration), the established norms may not be appropriate.

If, in the interest of time, you need to shorten your battery or your assessment package, the use of subscales may prove helpful; care, however, is needed in their selection. It is recommended that decisions such as these be based on empirical data. For example, you or other researchers may have found a subscale to be as good a predictor of outcome as the entire scale. In such a case you might decide to shorten your assessment battery by administering only that subscale. To take another example, if a split-half reliability test reveals comparable correlations between your measures of interest, you might decide to administer only the "odd" or "even" items of a lengthy scale, in the interest of time. While perhaps not "ideal," you have based your time-saving decisions on psychometrically sound principles.

Justification of Measures Selected

Keep the measurement section of the proposal brief, focused, and well justified. You should not simply state, "I want to measure depression." You need to explain how you want to measure depression (e.g., specify whether you are more concerned about prevalence of psychiatric disorders or the severity of their depressive symptoms). If you will be using qualitative approaches in assessing variables, this should be specified.

Citation for Instrument

For every instrument, cite the author and published source of the standardized instrument. Give the psychometric properties—the reliability and validity already established for this instrument. Discuss its use in the population that you are studying. (You will be on much better grounds if the measure you are using has already been used in that, or a similar, population.) Also, describe alternative measures and why you are not choosing them (e.g., "We are assessing AIDS-specific coping and we have looked at X, Y, and Z measures. Y and Z are inappropriate because . . . For these reasons, we are choosing X.") If you state your reasons, it will be very clear to the review committee that you have explored all your options and made your choices on a sound and rational basis. Include the actual instrument in your proposal's appendix and mention the modifications, if there are any.

Log of Measurement Decision

Keep a log about every research decision you make. If you change an instrument, write down when you did it, why, and with whom you consulted. It will be helpful later in documenting and reporting how and why the instrument became different from the original version. You will say, for example, "I used Beck's Hopelessness Scale, but instead of administering it in the usual manner, we administered it this way for X, Y, and Z reasons."

Summary: Strategy for Selecting Instruments

Steps to Be Taken

A. Identify your options

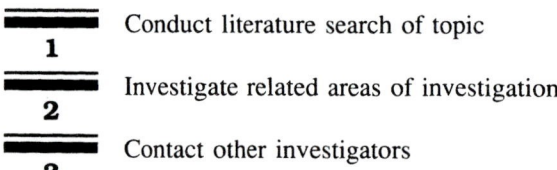

1 Conduct literature search of topic

2 Investigate related areas of investigation

3 Contact other investigators

B. Consider your resources and constraints

1 $$$

2 Determine time for assessment and study

3 Establish level of expertise of assessment personnel

4 Training and supervision

5 Population you will be studying

C. Establish criteria for choosing existing measures

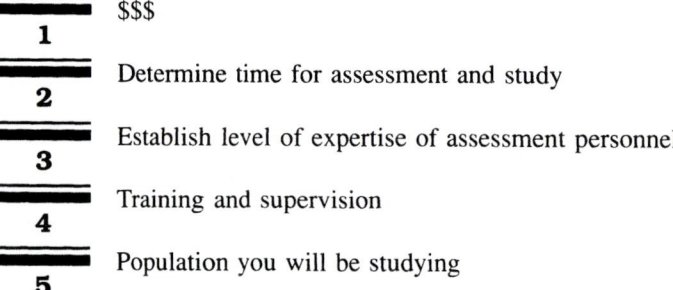

1 Write down constructs to be measured

2 Decide on mode of assessment (investigator-evaluated or self-report)

3 Preview standardized measures

4 Assess ability to evaluate your population with existing measures

D. Establish criteria for developing own measures

1 Inability to evaluate your population with own measures

2 Focus your study

Psychometric Issues

A. Basic properties to be considered

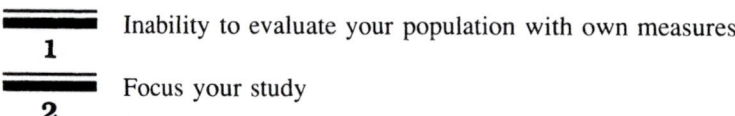

1 Reliability

2 Validity

B. Instrument modification and adaptation

    1 Changing items

    2 Adding items

    3 Eliminating items

    4 Using subscales

    5 Translation of measures

Grant Measurement Section

A. Description of measures should be brief and focused

B. What to include:

    1 Author and published references

    2 Psychometric properties

    3 Use in population to be studied

    4 Alternative measures and reasons for not selecting

    5 Training and supervision

C. Instruments should be included in appendix

Reference

Freeman, C., & Tyrer, P. 1989. *Research Methods in Psychiatry: A Beginner's Guide.* London: Gaskell, The Royal College of Psychiatrists (Distributed in North America by American Psychiatric Press, Inc.).

Additional Reading

Buros, O. C., ed. 1972. *The Seventh Mental Measurements Yearbook.* Highland Park, NJ: Gryphon Press.

Corcoran, K., & Fischer, J. 1987. *Measures for Clinical Practice: A Sourcebook.* New York: Free Press.

Huang K. H. C., Watters, J. K., & Case, P. 1988. Psychological assessment and AIDS research with intravenous drug users: Challenges in measurement. *Journal of Psychoactive Drugs 20:* 191–195.

Israel, L., Kozarenic, D., & Sartorius, N. 1984. *Source Book of Geriatric Assessment Volume 1: Evaluations in Gerontology.* New York: Karger.

Israel, L., Kozarenic, D., & Sartorius, N. 1984. *Source Book of Geriatric Assessment Volume 2: Review of Analyzed Instruments.* New York: Karger.

Lettieri, D. J., Nelson, J. E., & Sayers, M. A., eds. 1985. *NIAAA Treatment Handbook Series 2: Alcoholism Treatment Assessment Research Instruments.* Washington, DC: U.S. Government Printing Office.

Marsella, A. J., Hirschfeld, R. M. A., & Ratz, M. M., eds. 1987. *The Measurement of Depression.* New York: Guilford Press.

Rabkin, J. G. 1994. Self-rating scales for depression: Description and critique. Review prepared for the NIMH Depression Awareness, Treatment Program.

Van Riezen, H., & Segal, M. 1988. *Comparative Evaluations of Rating Scales for Clinical Psychopharmacology.* New York: Elsevier.

14

Integrating Psychological and Immunological Variables

Janice Kiecolt-Glaser

Many behavioral scientists planning to conduct research on HIV infection and AIDS may be wondering whether to include immunological measurement in your project. Generally, I recommend that you do not.

What often happens is that an investigator has interesting questions that may involve immunological data in only a tangential way. That person writes a proposal that asks good, straightforward research questions, but then tags on immunological measures. When the immunological measures are not well integrated into the study, this part is often reviewed poorly. The strengths of the study may be ignored because there are so many problems in the immunological arm of the study.

The lesson, then, is that if immunology is not a central focus of your study, be cautious about including immunological measures in your proposal; there are many ways that data collection and interpretation can become complicated. After all, immunological measures are not an essential component of most HIV studies that examine psychosocial variables. If, however, you feel that immunological data is important to answer your research questions, then you should carefully consider the following issues.

Selecting an Immunologist as a Collaborator

The first critical decision is selecting the appropriate immunologist with whom to collaborate. Without an immunologist's help, you will not have the necessary experience to deal with the inevitable methodological issues or to interpret the data. Most behavioral scientists are usually not competent to interpret immunological data.

In selecting an immunologist to work with, you should be aware that immunologists specialize more than behavioral scientists do. They have particular cells or subpopulations that they study. This raises the question, "What immunological measures should you include?" That may be the choice of your immunologist, because he or she may already be running those assays in his or her lab. While some assays are routine, many are complex, and it is not a simple matter to set up new assays. Thus, your immunologist may say that a measure you want to include is or is not possible within the available lab, timeframe, or budget.

Learning the Basics

Even if you are working with an immunologist, you should learn some basic immunology. For a psychologist or social scientist, it can be frustrating. Most medical school textbooks are unsatisfactory: "What is an antibody? Something that is stimulated by an antigen." "What is an antigen? Something that stimulates antibody production." Tautological explanations do not contribute to an understanding of the process.

If you want some basic immunology, which is a good idea for anyone working in the AIDS area, obtain an undergraduate microbiology text and read the two or three chapters on immunology. These books tend to be clearly written, and they will give you enough background so that you can read more advanced books, if necessary.

What to Measure

There are two general ways to assess immunological measures: (1) counting the number of immune cells and (2) evaluating how the cells function. In HIV infection, helper T-cell numbers are one of the markers of disease progression. With non–HIV-infected individuals, helper cells may change under stress, but it sometimes depends on the population, and so this is not a reliable measure.

Qualitative or functional aspects of immunity—how well cells function when exposed to a challenge or function—do appear to change with stress. For example, natural killer cell activity, an antiviral and antitumor defense, is one of the more reliable functions compromised by stress. Blastogenesis, which measures how lymphocytes proliferate when they are exposed to a substance called mitogen, is thought to provide a window for how lymphocytes proliferate when exposed to a pathogen, such as a virus or a bacteria.

When you choose your immunological assays, keep in mind that there are certain measures, noted in the psychoimmunological or immunological literature, that seem to change with stress and others that do not. These problems are compounded by HIV infection. With non–HIV-infected individuals, numbers of cells are not particularly stress responsive, while the functions of cells—natural killer cell activity, response to blastogenesis, lymphokine production—are more responsive to stressors.

Lymphokines, chemical mediators that stimulate immune function, tend to be depressed during stress. If you want to examine the relationship between stress and immune function, you may want to include both classes of assays if you have the resources. There is no single measure of immune function that gives you a measure of how the immune system is functioning, any more than there is a single measure of personality. The problem, then, is how to choose the measures to use in your study. For HIV, your single best measure is probably helper T-cells, but it would also be desirable to have other measures.

Cost

There is also the matter of cost. Immunological assays are expensive. If you look at hospital lab costs for helper T-cell assays, the costs of tests can range from $50 to more than $200 a test, depending on your area of the country. At that price, an immunological measure should make a substantial contribution to your study.

Interpreting Data

In addition to how and what to measure there are also some considerations that may affect how your immunological data is interpreted.

Time of Blood Draw

You will need to draw blood from all individuals in a given study within the same two-hour period. There is diurnal variation in the immune system that may be related to compartmentalization. Thus, if you draw blood from some subjects at 10 a.m., some at noon, some at 2 p.m., and some at 4 p.m., those individuals may well have very different baseline immune function that relates solely to the time of day at which their blood was drawn.

There is also evidence showing that the amount of time blood sits before you conduct the assay makes a difference. So the lab will need to be able to conduct the assays in a timely fashion.

Age

When you are looking at an immunological assay for your particular population, you need to be aware of your particular sample. The age of your study population is an important consideration. After puberty, the immune system declines; those declines are most pronounced among older adults. For people over 75 years of age, for example, pneumonia and influenza are together the fourth-leading cause of death. By and large, younger people who are not HIV-infected do not usually die of pneumonia and influenza.

Drug History

Some of the immunological data suggest that if people have a history of intravenous drug use, even if they are now clean, their immune function at base line is often worse. If you have a sample that is mixed in terms of individuals with prior or current injection drug use and no prior use, you will have a population that differs substantially in immunological functioning at base line that may be unrelated to your research question.

Another confounding factor is alcohol and illegal drug use, which certainly has an adverse effect on immune function. If you have a population that is abusing drugs, you will certainly have impaired immune function. This is important data to gather, even though it is not clear how those effects may be mediated.

This confound can even extend to caffeine and cigarette use, since there is some data suggesting that both caffeine and cigarette use may alter immune function. Caffeine may only produce transient effects, like giving someone a shot of epinephrine. Cigarette smoking, both direct and passive, may both be related to lower immune function, so you want to know what proportion of your sample smokes.

Medication Use

You have selected your immunological assays, a nutritional assessment, a measure of health-related behaviors, and then encounter a major confound: medication use. In some ways, the best individuals to study if we want to understand stress, health, and immune function are those who are going to be ill or who are already ill (i.e., HIV-infected individuals). However, HIV-infected individuals take a number of prescription and nonprescription medication, everything from megavitamin doses to AZT. Disentangling the effects of the medications from immune function when all of them may be immunoreactive is a major problem. The best way may be to have an adequate sample size so that you can control it statistically. You could use a control group of persons not taking any medication, but they would be more healthy than the experimental group and may differ in other ways that you could not control. For example, a larger percentage of older people take beta-blockers or estrogen. If you select only those who do not take medication, you are selecting survivors who may have abnormally active immune systems. In fact, one study that looked at unmedicated older individuals found that immune function appeared to increase with age, in contrast to the bulk of the immunological literature.

Health-Related Behaviors

One of the most important—and most often overlooked—problems will be the health-related behaviors that co-vary with stress (Kiecolt-Glaser & Glaser, 1988a). If a person is stressed, depressed, or upset in some way, they do things differently than people who are not. They are likely to eat more poorly, for example, and poor nutrition has adverse effects on immune function. Assessing nutritional status, however, is not an easy matter, and you will often end up doing quick measures (e.g., recent weight loss, normal range for height and weight, and perhaps plasma protein markers) that are not perfect, but are certainly better than nothing. With individuals who are already HIV-infected, there are concurrent nutritional changes that may also be taking place. These may be related to the infection, so it is important to be aware of what is happening in terms of nutrition.

Infection Illness

If you are assessing physical health and immune function, you want to know something about infectious illness in your subjects. This is one of the most difficult things to measure well because most physical health assessments look for global types of symptoms (e.g., malaise, fatigue, stomach aches). Those measures do not specifically relate to infectious illness. One of the batteries for measuring infectious illness is a health review that was developed for a study of air traffic controllers (Rose *et al.*, 1982a, b, c).

Final Thoughts

The key question is whether a relationship between psychological variables, actual changes in immune function, and illness exists. We now have good evidence for this relationship, albeit preliminary (Cohen *et al.*, 1991; Glaser *et al.*, 1992; Kiecolt-Glaser *et al.*, 1991).

The fact that stress can have adverse effects on immune function has been shown in a number of studies in both humans and other animals. If immune function is poor, a person's susceptibility to illness is much greater, especially with HIV. Anytime the immune system is suppressed radically, illness is more prolonged and more serious.

However, there is a paucity of data demonstrating the confluence of all three of those factors in the same individuals at the same time. That is important, because in most studies it is not possible to control whether someone becomes infected or not, nor can the dose of the pathogen be controlled. Therefore with semi-random patterns of infection, it is much harder to establish what is going on.

If you are not dissuaded, and you still want to include immunological measures in your behavioral study; that is good, because some of the stress/immune function data are among the most exciting. They have the potential to inform us about how stress, personal relationships, and health may be interrelated, and your well-designed study may make an important contribution (Kiecolt-Glaser & Glaser, 1988b).

References

Cohen, S., Tyrrell, D. A., & Smith, A. P. 1991. Psychological stress in humans and susceptibility to the common cold. *New England Journal of Medicine 325:* 606–612.

Glaser, R., Kiecolt-Glaser, J. K., Bonneau, R., Malarkey, W., & Hughes, J. 1992. Stress-induced modulation of the immune response to recombinant hepatitis B vaccine. *Psychosomatic Medicine 54:* 22–29.

Kiecolt-Glaser, J. K., & Glaser, R. 1988a. Methodological issues in behavioral immunology research with humans. *Brain, Behavior, and Immunity 2:* 67–78.

Kiecolt-Glaser, J. K., & Glaser, R. 1988b. Psychological influences on immunity: Implications for AIDS. *American Psychologist 43:* 892–898.

Kiecolt-Glaser, J. K., Dura, J. R., Speicher, C. E., Trask, O. J., & Glaser, R. 1991. Spousal caregivers of dementia victims: Longitudinal changes in immunity and health. *Psychosomatic Medicine 53:* 345–362.

Rose, R. M., Jenkins, C. D., Hurst, M., Livingston, L., & Hall, R. P. 1982a. Endocrine activity in air traffic controllers at work: I. Characterization of cortisol and growth hormone levels during the day. *Psychoneuroendocrinology 7:* 101–111.

Rose, R. M., Jenkins, C. D., Hurst, M., Herd, J. A., & Hall, R. P. 1982b. Endocrine activity in air traffic controllers at work: II. Biological, psychological and work correlates. *Psychoneuroendocrinology 7:* 113–123.

Rose, R. M., Jenkins, D. C., Hurst, M., Kreger, B. E., Barrett, J., & Hall, R. P. 1982c. Endocrine activity in air traffic controllers at work: III. Relationship to physical and psychiatric morbidity. *Psychoneuroendocrinology 7:* 125–134.

15

Institutional Review Boards and Special Human Subjects Issues in AIDS Research[1]

Judith Godwin Rabkin

Sources of IRB Regulations

Institutional Review Boards (IRBs) were first mandated by the federal government in 1974. The initial regulations have been revised and amended in successive years, most recently in 1991. These regulations technically cover only federally funded research involving the participation of human subjects. In practice, however, they apply to *all* research, because institutions sponsoring research do not like to have two sets of standards depending on funding source.

IRBs were established to prevent exploitation and deception in research (see Table 1 for central concepts). Central concepts in the federal regulations concern the provision of informed consent, so that potential subjects are given the information that most people would consider necessary to make a reasoned decision about research participation. Subjects must be informed about both the risks and benefits of the proposed research, about procedures the investigators will take to minimize the potential risks, and about how confidentiality is handled and what financial incentives, if any, are involved. In addition, IRBs pay careful attention to procedures for research recruitment. Subjects must be informed that their participation is voluntary; that is, they always reserve the option to decline research participation or withdraw at any time, without loss of benefits to which they are otherwise entitled. While the regulations cover many other issues, these are among the most salient to AIDS research.

[1] Editors' note: Although this chapter does not appear first in this section, it is really one of the most critical. Because AIDS applications are on an expedited review, IRB approval must be obtained *prior* to submission. If Block 4 on the cover sheet is not checked in the affirmative, the IRG cannot review your application. If there are extenuating circumstances, you should seek the advice of the Science Research Administrator (SRA) of the IRG to which you think your application will be referred prior to admission.

```
┌─────────────────────────────────────┐
│   Table 1. Central Concepts         │
│      in the Protection of           │
│        Human Subjects               │
│                                     │
│   Informed consent                  │
│   Risks and benefits                │
│   Minimizing potential risks        │
│   Confidentiality                   │
│   Financial incentives              │
│   Research recruitment              │
│   Voluntary participation           │
└─────────────────────────────────────┘
```

Although the federal regulations are detailed, they are flexible and give local IRBs considerable discretionary power. For example, there are special regulations for children's participation in research. Federal guidelines do not permit children to participate in research that is not intended for their direct benefit, when "the research involves more than a minor increment over minimal risk." This sounds very specific, but those words are not defined in the regulations. People disagree about the definitions of both minimal risk and minor increment. Thus, there is room for differing interpretations among IRBs at various institutions.

Flexibility in the federal guidelines has the advantage of allowing local standards to influence the action of local IRBs. The disadvantage to you is that the NIMH grant review committee may not agree with your IRB and may raise human subjects concerns even if you have local IRB approval. This difference of opinion must then be brought to the attention of your IRB.

For grant applications, the only IRB approval that must be obtained in advance is that of the institution sponsoring the research, even if more than one institution is involved. It is customary for the sponsoring IRB to give provisional approval, and, after funding is assured, other necessary approvals can be obtained and then final IRB approval can be granted. The same applies to obtaining a Certificate of Confidentiality, which is discussed below.

There is usually more than one regulatory agency involved in telling the IRBs, and therefore you, what can or cannot be done. Federal regulations apply to all of us, but states often have laws or regulations that govern research. For example, in federal regulations there is a category of research that is "exempt," but New York State's mental hygiene law says no research is exempt. Therefore, New York's IRBs do not use that category. In addition to federal and state laws, all drug trials are subject to FDA regulations. Universities and hospitals also may have guidelines for protection of research participants.

There may be another complication as well. If you are working with more than one institution in AIDS research—it is very common that you are affiliated with a community agency, a hospital, and a university—each may have an IRB. You can end up, then, having several agencies telling you what to do.

Easing Your Way through the IRB

In AIDS research, unlike other areas of research, IRB approval has to arrive *with* your grant application; in all other areas of research, you have a 60-day grace period to submit the IRB approval after the grant deadline. Because of the expedited review cycle for AIDS grants, the Science Research Administrators (SRA) must have IRB approval prior to assigning your research application to a reviewer.

Sometimes this is a problem for investigators, and exceptions of a week or so may be obtained from the SRA, but advance planning is clearly needed. Of course, the best way to avoid this problem is to initiate the IRB approval process two months in advance. Unfortunately, most investigators do not have their grant applications finished two months in advance to send to the IRB for review. There are ways, though, to ease this process.

Find out the meeting schedule of your IRB. Some meet monthly, while others meet only when needed. Understand that there are some issues that are more important than others for IRBs. They are not supposed to be scientific review committees, although sometimes it is a fine distinction since their task is to weigh the risks and benefits of the proposed research, which often entails an evaluation of scientific merit. For example, the feasibility of your recruitment plan is less salient than the actual procedures of how you recruit your subjects; the latter can be a sensitive issue, especially in AIDS research.

Informed Consent

IRBs need a detailed description of informed consent procedures; as a matter of fact, review committees are also interested. You are not required to include a consent form with your grant, but a lucid consent form can help the reviewer to understand what you are going to do from the subject's point of view, what you ascertain are the risks and benefits, and how you present them to potential research subjects.

The standard procedure is to obtain written consent, although IRBs have some discretionary power. For example, if you are going to conduct an anonymous telephone survey, you cannot obtain written consent. In most other instances, if you are in a face-to-face situation, it makes sense to have a written document. Sometimes, though, the investigator should sign the consent form because it may be more of a risk to the subject to have his or her name on a consent form retained in your files than it is not to have documentation of consent. For example, a child psychiatrist in our department planned to interview adolescent street hustlers on the waterfront. The investigator did not need identifying information for research purposes. Since he was

---

Table 2. Features of Your Consent Form That Facilitate Approval

Provide a clear statement about the purpose of the study.

Write it in language appropriate for the educational level of your proposed subjects.

Make an effort to write your consent form in simple English. This is important because the educational level of your subjects may only be at the seventh or eighth grade. If English is the second language for your subjects, this will help ensure that they understand the study. Avoid jargon, use short sentences, and organize the material with subheadings to make it easier to follow.

Use a reader-friendly format with reasonable margin, spacing, and font size.

Discuss the study procedures from the subject's vantage point—where will the study take place, how long will it take, what exactly will the procedure entail, etc.

Describe risks and benefits and procedures for risk minimization.

Explain payments, if any. Payments are not a benefit of research, because the way the federal regulations are written, the benefit is supposed to be a direct consequence of the research participation. Money is an incentive.

If you are conducting a treatment study, you need to describe alternative treatments if there are any.

collecting information about criminal behavior, having subjects sign consent forms itself posed a risk to them. Instead, the IRB proposed that the investigator read the consent form to each participant, answer any questions, and himself sign the form to indicate that the consent process had been executed.

An important thing to remember about consent forms is that they are not the place for a hard sell, particularly if more than minimal risk is involved. Be conservative and modest in tone. It is rare for someone to read a consent form and then back out.

There is an important category in an informed consent form called "Research Standards and Rights of Participants." This is where you answer questions concerning the regulations and guidelines having to do with voluntary participation, the right to withdraw without loss of benefits to which subjects are otherwise entitled, how to obtain a copy of the consent form, how to know the consent form was approved by an IRB and so forth. See Table 2 for more information on consent forms.

Confidentiality

Confidentiality is always an important consideration for IRBs, but in AIDS research it assumes a central role. Given prevailing levels of stigma and discrimination toward persons with HIV illness, protection of confidentiality is crucial. The best way to handle this issue is not to collect any identifying information. If you see research participants only once and do not need to link any records, do not ask them for any identifying information. This also applies to surveys or single-occasion interviews.

When conducting a treatment study or any longitudinal research where data are collected multiple times, it is necessary to link data over time. One method to ensure confidentiality is to give the subject complete responsibility for identifying himself/herself with a code number on each occasion. For example, they could use the last four digits of their social security number or some combination of personal data. The problem is the risk of error, especially in a population where cognitive impairment may become manifest with illness progression.

When you must collect some identifying information from study participants in order to track them, you often need less than is initially expected. For example, some grant offices routinely require that subjects provide Social Security numbers when paid for research. This turns out to be a negotiable requirement, and exceptions can be made. Another way to protect confidentiality of serostatus is to include some HIV seronegative subjects in a protocol for subjects with HIV illness; otherwise simply being a study participant would reveal an individual's serostatus. Is the study conducted in a geographically distinct area so that all subjects seen there are necessarily in an HIV protocol? Do you need to collect identifying information about sexual partners? (This is particularly important to think about in states requiring contact tracing.) Overall, the guiding principle should be to avoid collecting identifying information to the extent possible, since you cannot report to authorities what you do not know.

If you decide that you must collect identifying information, a method now widely used in AIDS research is to obtain from the federal government a Certificate of Confidentiality. While this is not an absolute guarantee of confidentiality, it is perhaps the best available protection. A Certificate of Confidentiality protects the investigator from involuntary disclosure of identifying information regarding research participants. You must also provide assurance of confidentiality to your study participants; you must promise them that no member of the research team will divulge voluntarily identifying information. You should have all the people on your staff sign an agreement to that effect. Having this Certificate means that you are not obliged to release identifying information about research participants to any federal, state, or local administrative, legislative, or executive body. If you are served with a subpoena, you do not have to respond. This has been in effect for over 15 years and has never been challenged in court.

Although the absence of a challenge is reassuring, it also means that there is no case law to support a

Certificate of Confidentiality. In theory, federal certificates supersede state and local laws. However, one should be extremely careful about taking that literally, because usually the state and local laws it supersedes include reporting child abuse, suicidal or homicidal intent, or other things that you might seriously consider making an exception to in a promise of confidentiality. This is particularly relevant with adolescents and other potentially risky populations.

There is a fine line to draw between being a scientist and a citizen. For example, a study conducted in our institution is with runaways who are in a shelter, but they may leave and engage in risky behaviors on the street, and they may sell drugs to each other. At what point are you obliged to report this behavior, to whom do you report it, and what behavior do you have to report? There are no simple answers to these questions.

You should consider applying for a Certificate of Confidentiality if identifying participants in your study might pose a risk to them, which is frequently the case in AIDS research. It only takes ½ hour to write a letter, and you have to do it about six to eight weeks before you actually begin the study. You must obtain a separate certificate for each study.

As noted, the Certificate of Confidentiality does not prevent you from disclosing information voluntarily; it just means that you cannot be forced to do so. You can release information voluntarily if you think it is clinically indicated. But it is prudent to advise people initially, in the process of informed consent, the exact limits of your promise of confidentiality.

A final point about confidentiality has to do with the grant review committees. If you are working with a population where confidentiality is an issue, it is helpful to reviewers to be explicit about how you are going to maintain confidentiality of data on questionnaires during data management and analysis. Be specific, for example, about who will have access to the data and the computers and what procedures you intend to use to limit access.

Human Subjects and the Grant Application

Remember that Section E of the grant application, the one directed to the protection of human subjects, is not included in the 20-page limit. In general, reviewers appreciate brevity in every aspect of the grant application, but this section gives you an opportunity to expand upon some of the areas that you may not have had room to cover adequately in the earlier part of the application.

This is the place to describe exactly who your subjects will be, what the criteria are for inclusion and exclusion, what risk minimization procedures you are going to observe, and how you define the criteria for study participation. For example, if one of the criteria for inclusion is good physical health, describe in Section E how you will operationalize this concept and measure it.

Financial Incentives

This is also the section where you need to describe incentives you propose to use in recruiting participants. This is particularly relevant for working with communities where research is not a standard value. When you are working in minority communities, for example, it may not be prevailing norm to be altruistic about research participation, and sometimes you have to provide incentives or inducements that you might not have to in other circumstances.

Federal guidelines say that you should not pay people more money than they otherwise earn in their usual occupation. One problem is that there is differential renumeration for the same effort. Another problem in adhering to this guideline is that the reimbursement rate is difficult to define if your subjects are not currently working.

There is another matter concerning incentives. It is permitted to pay people to be bored, but it is not acceptable to pay people to take risks. If your study involves risks—taking an investigational drug, for example—you should not pay for research participation. If you are going to administer a 4-hour family history and individual psychiatric evaluation, the only risk is that the subject will be bored, but it is permissible to pay.

If more than one session is involved, you should not pay at the end, because that is coercion. Otherwise the subject really is not free to withdraw from research participation because all payment will be sacrificed. Worse, subjects who get sick because of study participation and drop out for this reason are deprived of payment. So you should prorate the incentive. You can give a balloon payment as a reward for finishing the entire study, but participants must be given something along the way so that they can decide to quit without losing out entirely.

Mandatory Reporting of HIV Test Results to Subjects

If you do HIV testing as part of your project and you receive federal funds for the project, federal regulations require that you report the results of the HIV test to your study participants. They do not have the option of *not* hearing the results if they are going to stay in a research study funded by the federal government. You therefore must provide pre- and post-counseling to everybody in the study, even if the results are negative. The regulations do not, however, specify a time period within which subjects must be informed of their HIV status. This does not apply if you blind seroprevalence tests; for example, if you use anonymous blood samples that have only code numbers and general information like age, gender, and ethnicity and blood samples are sent to the laboratory in batches, you cannot inform subjects of their individual results.

Release of Research Data to Third Parties

Participants are concerned about release of sensitive data to third parties, and, in such cases, Certificates of Confidentiality and written agreements by investigators not to release data voluntarily are reassuring. Sometimes, research participants ask investigators to inform others of their HIV test or laboratory test results (e.g., to facilitate getting government benefits, to save the cost of redundant tests). There may be concern that subjects may be under pressure from others to make such requests or that the authorized "others" really should not be recipients of such information. One solution we have found helpful is to refuse to release any sensitive information to anyone over the phone but to hand deliver copies of test results to research subjects.

Summary

Although it is often disheartening to contemplate more paperwork and regulations when one is in the process of completing a grant application, IRB review is not only necessary but can also be helpful. It requires you to think about the logistics and details of your procedures and, surprisingly, often leads to a strengthening of your research design. Considering the research from the participants' point of view can provide new insights and perspectives that may be to your advantage as well as to the advantage of your research subjects.

16

Developing a Résumé and Presenting a Staff

Leonard Mitnick

In every NIMH Program Announcement or Request for Applications there is a section entitled "Review Criteria." A major review criterion is the research experience and competence of the Principal Investigator (PI) and the research team to conduct the proposed research project. Specific issues are the demonstrated expertise of the PI and key personnel, adequacy of the effort devoted to the project, schedule of activities proposed, and staff coverage.

Research Partners

Currently much research that is being conducted is interdisciplinary, and this is particularly true of AIDS research. Thus, it is important to assemble a team that reflects the expertise required to perform your project. Do not add people with different skills and different disciplines without a rationale. For example, if your outcome measures involve immunological assays, you will need an immunologist who has a lab prepared to do that specific work. Do not hire the chairman of a department who has not been in a laboratory for 10 years to do an assay that requires current laboratory expertise. If you are planning to develop instruments, you will need someone who can establish their reliability and validity. An anthropologist may be essential if an ethnographic study is proposed as part of your multimethod study. If you do not have those skills, make sure that someone on your research team does and that the biographical sketch demonstrates that expertise.

There are four places in the Public Health Service Form 398 (Rev. 9/91) to describe the competence of the research team responsible for the scientific development and conduct of the study. On page 2, you list the key personnel, project roles, and affiliation. Page 4 of the budget gives proposed level of effort for major personnel on the project. Under the "Personnel" section you can highlight the specific areas of responsibility for the major persons. Finally, a two-page "Biographical Sketch" is included for the key personnel.

Key Personnel

While there can only be one PI, key personnel are colleagues who will devote major effort to this project and will have responsibilities during the entire grant period. They will often assume roles as Co-PIs or co-investigators. Key personnel are usually at the same institution as the PI.

Consultants

In addition to key personnel, you may also need consultants who will have a much more narrow and defined role, such as in the areas of experimental design or data analysis. Consultants provide critical but often relatively brief consultation on a research project. At points they can review the way an intervention is being conducted, interpret results from immunological assays, or provide expert advice on the conduct of data analysis. Describe the skills and expertise they possess that make them essential for your study. You have to state why you are bringing a consultant in for a short period of time, and you have to explain the specific task that they are going to perform for you.

Allocation of Effort

Consider carefully the percent of time that each person will spend on the project. Some applicants think, "I'm going to get a well-known expert and put him or her down for 5 percent of full time." Five percent translates to approximately 2 hours a week, which may not be adequate for the contribution that is required of the person. On the other hand, you may only need a person for a specific task at designated times during the project. If the hours that this task takes turn out to be 5 percent, state that clearly with the rationale.

A review committee examining the budget page and seeing 5 percent allocated to many people may ask, "Who is conducting the research?" You must describe who is responsible for each part of the project. If you do not have the money to hire someone, ask a specific colleague for a commitment contingent on funding. This person should provide a letter indicating willingness to collaborate on the study, and a current curriculum vitae (CV) should be included so his/her expertise can also be evaluated.

Professional Experience

In completing the "Biographical Sketch" be sure to comply with the 2-page limitation in the section on professional experience. Conclude with your present position and list your previous employment experience in chronological order. Include any honors and memberships on committees that are relevant to a research career.

If you are in your first position as an assistant professor in charge of research and evaluation, describe your responsibilities. Indicate the courses that you teach, your areas of research interests, your research honors, and other information that relates to your research competence. In this context, it is not an honor that a local radio station interviewed you about your opinions on some issue.

Publications

List in chronological order the titles and complete references to all publications during the past three years and representative earlier publications pertinent to this application.

A publication is an article that has been accepted in a refereed journal. You want the reviewers to see some demonstration of your research competence. It is acceptable to include publications "in press," but an article submitted for publication does not carry weight, however, because it has not yet been peer reviewed. If you have the space, list a publication even if you are the third or fourth author. A section entitled "Work in Progress" at the end of your résumé is also acceptable. If there are no relevant publications to this application, you may say so.

If you have changed research areas, you may have 10 or 15 publications from five years ago in an area unrelated to your current project, but only a few in the past few years related to your new area of research. You may list a few of the older articles in the journals that are the most highly respected scientifically in order to demonstrate that you have had a research career and a research history.

List book chapters separately from journal articles, because books or chapters are secondary sources. They are acceptable, and it is important that you have been asked to write a chapter, but often they have not been peer reviewed and do not carry the same weight.

You should also list abstracts that have been presented at a competitive conference and published in an abstract book. If you have prepared a poster, this is important, because in many AIDS meetings posters are the only format for presenting new data.

Assessing Your Résumé

When you have completed your research resume ask yourself, "Will this statement communicate my research competence and ability to conduct the proposed study to the review committee?" If you have a positive response, ask a colleague to review your "Biographical Sketch" and see if he or she concurs. As the PI you should also critically review the résumé of each person on your project.

Concluding Comments

The research expertise of the PI and key personnel is a critical factor in receiving a positive review of the proposal. Do not send an old résumé or a photocopy because that reflects negatively upon you. Take the time to be sure that the four sections where you can provide information on the expertise and level of effort of your team are well integrated and adequately present documentation of the skills required to conduct the proposed study.

17

Developing the Data Analytic Plan

H. Gerry Taylor

Introduction and Aims

Preparing grant applications is a difficult and anxiety-laden process for everyone. The problems we face and the obstacles we must overcome for successful grantsmanship are similar, whatever our area of interest or theoretical bent. Although the primary aim of this chapter is to discuss components of the data analytic section of a grant proposal, my larger purpose is to review the grant-writing process more generally. It is impossible to write a competitive data analytic section without having first developed a sound rationale and appropriate study design. The data analytic section provides necessary details regarding data analytic plan, but this section will only make sense if the applicant has already set forth a clear and defensible rationale, formulated testable hypotheses, attended to potential methodological pitfalls, proposed an appropriate study design, and convinced the reviewer that the study is both novel and feasible.

The data analytic section is, in a sense, the "final common pathway" for the idea being proposed. More than any other section, it gives the reviewer an overview of the researcher's conceptual and methodological talents and of the likelihood that the study will be properly conducted.[1] This section also helps the reviewer answer many of the questions that will be critical in rating the proposal:

✔ Will findings be scientifically meaningful?

✔ Does the researcher have a good grasp of the need for operational definitions of concepts?

✔ Will data sets be properly managed?

[1] Editors' note: Many reviewers feel that it should be possible to derive the study by reading the data analytic plan.

✔ Are plans for analysis reasonable given current statistical methods and the types of measures involved, and are new findings likely to emerge?

Affirmative answers to these questions require that the entire proposal be well thought out.

My personal experience with the grant-writing process has been in seeking federal support for research in the area of developmental neuropsychology and as a reviewer serving on grant review committees. I have learned that there is consensus among reviewers with regard to the prerequisites for a good grant application. My impressions are that most criticisms of grant applications can be classified into six categories: (1) general considerations, (2) design and hypothesis, (3) subjects, (4) measures, (5) data analytic plan, and (6) experimental treatments. Under each category, I have posed questions commonly asked by reviewers which you should ask yourself as you review your proposal.

General Considerations

1 Is the proposal driven by a theory or central set of questions or hypotheses?

2 Is the idea important and original?

3 Is the rationale clear, meaningful, and well conceptualized?

4 Is the proposal written in an acceptable format, and is it well organized?

5 Is the proposal focused and clear as to what the priority issues are, or is it expansive and overly ambitious?

6 Are the hypotheses testable, and is the proposal explicit as to how they will be tested?

7 Does the proposal indicate that the researchers are knowledgeable about the issues under investigation, and are appropriate co-investigators and consultants involved?

8 Have the applicants considered limitations and potential problems? Do they indicate how they will deal with these problems, and are their choices convincing?

9 Are strengths also evident?

10 Does the proposal reflect a process of "thinking through" the issues under investigation from the available research literature to testable hypotheses, operational measurement, anticipated results, and interpretation of alternative findings?

11 Are new and significant findings likely to emerge (applied and/or theoretical), and will the study expand the existing knowledge base?

12 Do methods or theories have broader applications to other conditions?

13 Are study aims and procedures culturally sensitive and ethically acceptable?

14 Are members of the research team qualified to do the study, and do they work in a supportive environment?

15 Is the proposed budget appropriate, and are costs justified?

Design and Hypotheses

1   Is the design clearly presented?

2   Is the design defensible in terms of sensitivity to processes under study, feasibility, experimental control, and statistical precision?

3   Are the hypotheses explicit and testable?

4   Has previous work (e.g., related research or pilot research) been conducted to document the validity of the measures, study feasibility, and the credibility of the hypotheses?

5   Has subject attrition been considered?

6   Are manipulations of independent variables potent enough to result in changes in the dependent variables?

7   Have confounding factors been considered so that the results will be interpretable (i.e., relate to the process of interest)?

8   Are sampling strategies and measurement methods replicable?

9   Will findings be generalizable, and what conclusions will be drawn?

Subjects

1   Are criteria for inclusion and exclusion of subjects clear and complete?

2   Is recruitment feasible?

3   Is the sample adequately described?

4   Is the sample representative of the population of interest?

5   Have detection (referral) biases been considered?

Measures

1   Are independent and dependent variables and covariates clearly specified?

2   Are constructs adequately defined?

3   Have the reliability and validity of the measures been adequately established in previous work?

4 Will measures be sensitive and comprehensive enough to provide for adequate test of the hypotheses?

5 Is response burden too heavy for the participants?

6 Are means available to help establish the validity of subjective, or self-report, measures (e.g., attempts to consensually validate the measures and to take response sets such as social desirability into account)?

7 Have all other sources of measurement bias been considered (e.g., testers blind to group membership, recall or response bias, common method variance)?

8 If repeated testing is proposed, are measures susceptible to practice effects or reactivity, and what is the researcher's plan for dealing with these troublesome issues?

9 Are clinical disorders well defined, and are clinical correlates being examined?

Data Analytic Plan

1 Does the analytic plan correspond to the hypotheses?

2 Are statistical procedures appropriate, and are methods for testing hypotheses sufficiently detailed?

3 Are there ways to summarize multivariate outcomes (e.g., factor scores, summary variables) that would help to minimize the number of dependent variables?

4 How will Type I error be minimized to take multiple comparisons into account?

5 In cases of multiple comparisons, are there also plans for controlling Type II error (e.g., grouping of dependent variables on a conceptual basis)?

6 Is the proposed sample size justified by power calculations?

7 Does the research team possess the necessary expertise to ensure appropriate handling of complex statistical issues (e.g., statisticians, experts in analytic methods)?

Experimental Treatments

1 Is there good reason to expect that the proposed treatment will be efficacious?

2 Is there a clear rationale for choice of the comparison group (e.g., to rule out spontaneous recovery as an explanation for observed treatment effects, to establish the mechanisms responsible for these effects, or to isolate the "active" component of a treatment program)?

3 Is the treatment well described?

4 How can the researchers ensure that subjects will be motivated to perform treatment activities and that the treatment has achieved its stated goals (i.e., has resulted in increased knowledge or skills)?

5 How will the fidelity of the treatment be maintained across settings, therapists, and time?

6 Is there a possibility that the effects of the experimental manipulation will "spill over" into the comparison group(s) (e.g., through informal conversations of study participants)?

7 Have other possible contaminants been considered (e.g., alternative treatments from others or self-learning of other methods)?

8 Are there plans to assess both immediate and longer-term effects of treatment?

9 Have potential measurement biases been considered (e.g., desirability, expectancies)?

10 Has attrition been taken into account?

11 Are there plans to assess variables that may predict individual treatment response (e.g., gender, age, social or educational background)?

A Model of an Excellent Grant Application

An example of a well-crafted research proposal is reproduced in Appendix A on page 191.[2] The data analytic section is appropriately thorough and is well integrated with the remainder of the proposal.

This proposal is a good case study in grantsmanship. Brief review of this proposal will show that it has responded effectively to most if not all of the major criteria listed in this chapter. Answers to checklist items are easily located; and, although the proposal does not have a treatment component, it demonstrates how one group of researchers successfully addressed critical issues in the development of a research application.

The proposal is clearly written and well organized. It addresses important issues in AIDS research with pediatric populations and provides a cogent review of the existing literature. What is most impressive is the way in which the study is framed around the major study aims and hypotheses. Other strengths include the inclusion of a methodological critique of past studies in the area, the extent to which potential methodological problems of the proposed project are anticipated, the sophistication evident in the treatment of covarying social factors, and the details provided with regard to feasibility, subjects, and measures.

One has the clear impression that the proposal is well reasoned, that the investigators are experienced and have problem-solved major methodological issues, and that new and useful findings are likely to emerge. The proposal also highlights information most essential to the reviewer. The experimental design is presented in a straightforward and summary manner at the beginning of the "Experimental

---

[2] The grant application is entitled "Neurodevelopmental Status in HIV Positive Ugandan Infants" (Karen Olness, M.D., Principal Investigator). The application received a favorable review and was funded by NIH. The proposal itself was an extension of a previously initiated study of the effects of HIV positivity on pregnancy and birth. It was designed to follow two groups of children born to the HIV-positive or HIV-negative mothers. The two primary comparisons of interest were between infants with and without HIV positivity (at birth and thereafter) and infected infants with and without clinical symptoms of AIDS. The essential aims of the proposal were threefold: (1) to determine the neurodevelopmental consequences of HIV infection in children from birth to 24 months of age, (2) to investigate the extent to which infant testing procedures are able to detect risks for later abnormalities, and (3) to study other influences on the child's development, such as nutritional status, maternal health, family demographics, and caretaking.

Design and Methods" section. Procedures for subject selection, recruitment, and laboratory testing are clearly indicated. Methods for solving measurement problems and for enhancing reliability and consistency are also noted. The outcome measures are divided into conceptually meaningful sets representing primary dependent variables and covariates, with the reader appropriately referred to appendices for more detailed descriptions of measures or for actual test protocols. Finally, the components of the proposal are clearly outlined. This makes it easy for the reviewer to understand the proposal and find answers to any specific questions.

Writing the Data Analytic Plan

The sections of this proposal that deal with data analysis, power calculations, and data management are particularly good examples of how to present data analytic plans. Because of page restrictions, applicants often condense their proposals, and some have chosen to provide only a minimum plan for data processing. The data analytic section of this model proposal, although not unduly detailed, demonstrates an awareness of statistical analysis and a plan for testing hypotheses.

The applicants specify procedures for data management and data reduction, and they appreciate the need for descriptive analyses. Examples include procedures for data input, age standardization, derivation of factor scores, and definition of variables summarizing language performance and nutritional status. They have plans for examining the frequency of abnormal outcomes as well as for comparisons of group means. Methods for hypothesis testing are described at some length, including identification of the major independent and dependent variables and specification of analytic procedures. The applicants also summarize plans for taking covariates into account, review sample attrition, and justify sample size by means of power calculations. The appropriateness of the plans and the participation of co-investigators with statistical expertise assures the reviewer that analyses will be conducted appropriately.

Of course, there are many ways to organize the data analytic section, and the proposal in Appendix A is only one example. Content and length will vary substantially with the area of investigation, the hypotheses to be tested, and complexity of the design and analysis. What is most critical is that this section be well integrated with the rest of the proposal and that it reflect a level of sophistication that will convince the reviewer that the applicants are knowledgeable about the appropriate methods and have thought through important problems. Central to each proposal is the need to communicate precisely how the hypotheses will be tested, to justify the sample size, and to address methodological and statistical complexities familiar to those who have conducted work in the field (i.e., the reviewers).

Experience in analyzing preliminary or related data sets is undoubtedly the best way to become familiar with these complexities. It is also helpful to consult with persons who have analyzed similar data sets. A sampling of the many excellent review articles and textbooks pertaining to methodological issues and statistical techniques is included in the "Additional Reading" section that follows. Hopefully, readers will find these resources, together with the checklist and appended proposal, constructive in writing their next grant or grant revision.

Additional Reading

Bock, R. D. 1975. *Multivariate Statistics for the Behavioral Sciences.* New York: McGraw-Hill.

Cohen, J. 1977. *Statistical Power Analyses for the Behavioral Sciences.* New York: Academic Press.

Cohen, J., & Cohen, P. 1983. *Multiple Regression/Correlational Analyses for the Behavioral Sciences.* Hillsdale, NJ: Erlbaum.

Feinstein, A. R. 1988. Scientific standards in epidemiologic studies of the menace of daily life. *Science 242:* 1257–1263.

Huberty, C. J., & Morris, J. D. 1989. Multivariate analysis versus multiple univariate analysis. *Psychological Bulletin 105 (2)*: 302–308.

Kleinbaum, D. G., Kupper, L. L., & Muller, K. E. 1988. *Applied Regression Analysis and Other Multivariate Methods* (2nd ed.). Boston: P.W.S. Kent.

O'Brien, R. G., & Kaiser, M. K. 1985. MANOVA method for analyzing repeated measure designs: An extensive primer. *Psychological Bulletin 97:* 316–333.

Schlesselman, J. J. 1982. *Case-Control Studies: Design, Conduct, Analysis.* New York: Oxford.

Tabachnick, B. G., & Fedell, L. S. 1983. *Using Multivariate Statistics.* New York: Harper & Row.

18

Developing a Budget and Financial Justification

Frank Mucha

Your research budget should clearly reflect resources needed for the proposed project, and it should be reasonable, believable, and superbly justified. Justify everything in the budget that may not be clear; the reviewers will be able to judge the merit of your hypotheses better if they do not have to solve mysteries.

It is helpful to justify budget items in the same sequence as they appear on the budget page. Each cost category—such as personnel, equipment, supplies, and travel—should clearly stand out as a subsection so that the reviewers may quickly and easily find the needed information.

Often applicants are not careful to specify budget changes in subsequent years. Make it clear that you are not trying to "sneak in" an unnecessary expense. Indicate and justify all substantial changes in the pattern of expenditures from year to year. The awarding Institute will allow a fixed percentage of increase on all recurring expenses. It is up to you to show, for instance, that the increase you are proposing is related to increased field activity or that your data will be so numerous in year 3 that you will have to double the data manager's effort.

Remember that the reviewers expect to find a clear and justifiable relation between the proposed project and the requested budget. The review of most applications does not include a site visit, which would give the applicant a chance to explain the ambiguities. Therefore you must make your proposal as clear, concise, and convincing as you can. Clarity and conciseness are not mutually exclusive. (See Appendix B, for which I am indebted to Mr. Fred Averick, on pages 217–228 for an example of completed budget pages and justification.)

Personnel

The following discussion addresses issues included on form pages 4 and 5 only (Detailed Budget page for initial budget period and Budget for entire proposed budget period). Note that there are different requirements for listing personnel on other pages.

List the names and roles of all applicant organization personnel involved in the project, whether or not salaries are requested. Do not list any personnel who are affiliated with consortium or third party institutions. All budget categories are to reflect the applicant organization's costs only. Consortium institutions will develop their own individual detailed budget pages to be included with the grantee's application.

Begin with the PI, and then list all key personnel followed by support personnel. One column describes the type of appointment, i.e., full-time, half-time academic, full-time summer, etc. The appointment is expressed in number of months. The next column indicates the percentage of each appointment devoted to this project and is expressed as a percentage.

Where funds are requested, the maximum salary that may be applied for is calculated by multiplying the individual's base salary by the percentage to be devoted to the project. If a lesser amount is requested for any position, explain the difference on page 5 of the application (for example, endowed position, institutional sources, RCDA, other support). Fringe benefits may be requested to the extent that they are treated consistently by the applicant as direct cost to all sponsors.

Personnel: Do Nots

✔ Do not forget to list yourself and your percentage of effort.

✔ Do not exceed 100% of the collective sum of percentages of time and effort proposed for each individual across all of their activities.

✔ Do not mix salaries with consulting fees.

✔ Do not include salaries of people not associated with your institution (unless the salary is to be paid through your institution). In such a case obtain a sign-off from the institution for which the person is working.

Questions Reviewers May Ask about Personnel

✔ Is the number of professional and nonprofessional staff consistent with the effort required by the research protocol?

✔ Does the amount requested for personnel to be appointed reflect anticipated beginning dates for such appointments?

✔ Are the requirements for some portions of the research protocol so extensive that they justify request for personnel that might otherwise be considered inflated?

✔ Is the time or effort allocated for each person consistent with other concurrent or pending efforts with which each may be involved?

✔ Does the budget reflect the time or effort for those who would be working on the project but who would receive total or partial renumeration from other sources of support?

✔ Does the budget include an appropriate request for fringe benefits, and does the institution allocate the fringe benefits to direct or indirect cost?

✔ Does the request reflect anticipated mid-year increases?

Consulting Costs

Give the name and institutional affiliation for any consultant involved in the proposed grant activity. If the consultant is an employee of the grantee institution, be sure to indicate that the consultation is across departmental lines and in addition to regular duties (or that it involves a separate or remote operation) and that the work performed is in addition to the consultant's regular departmental workload. In addition, you should show that the relevant Institution(s) is/are aware and approve of this arrangement. Be sure to itemize the costs of the consultant, including the rate compensation, per diem, travel, and other related costs. The base salary is the compensation that the applicant organization pays.

Consultants: Do Nots

- ✔ Do not request consultants that cannot be justified, either because of lack of expertise or inappropriate level of effort.
- ✔ Do not request consultants that cannot be justified by their potential contribution to the proposed research.
- ✔ Do not request consultants that have not agreed to participate.

Questions Reviewers May Ask about Consultants

- ✔ Who are the consultants?
- ✔ With what institutions are the consultants affiliated?
- ✔ Are the consultants so well known that biographical sketches are not needed?
- ✔ What portions of the project require advice from consultants?

Equipment

List separately each item with a unit requisition cost of $500 or more. Be sure to justify (page 5 of the application) the reasons for requesting items of equipment that appear to duplicate or to be equivalent to equipment listed on the Resources and Environment page. Since it is generally expected that the institution will ordinarily provide general-purpose equipment (office equipment and furnishings, heating and cooling units, passenger and cargo vehicles, computing and automatic data processing devices, cameras, etc.), any request for items of this nature should be specifically justified on page 5. The equipment category should be closely related to the later discussion of "Resources and Environment."

Equipment: Do Nots

- ✔ Do not ask for equipment that appears to be duplicative (for example, if the investigator requested such equipment in previous proposals).
- ✔ Do not assume that the need for any item is obvious.

Questions Reviewers May Ask about Equipment

- ✔ Are these items already available in the institution's inventory of unused equipment?
- ✔ Are these items available in nearby laboratories, and could they be shared?
- ✔ Would it be more economical to rent or lease any of the items rather than purchase them?

Supplies

Itemize supplies in separate categories, such as $X for glassware, $Y for chemicals etc., although categories in amounts less than $1,000 do not have to be itemized. If animals are involved, state the number to be used, their unit purchase costs, and their unit care cost. Show calculations of the cost of supplies for assays, individual tests, and other procedures. Use charts and time lines, and make sure that your calculations correspond with the chronology and logistics of the scientific text (number and timing of testing of subjects, animals, etc. (See Appendix C on pages 229–242 for an excellent example of time lines and charts.)

In calculating the cost of supplies (also technical services, tests, assays, etc.), quantification that relates directly to the population tested, assays to be done, and interviewer's time needed is a necessity. It is important, however, to find the middle road so that the reviewer is not inundated by calculations. One should not lose sight of the forest while concentrating on the trees.

Supplies: Do Nots

✔ Do not request supplies indiscriminately.

✔ Do not use animal species that cannot be correlated to human data or are not appropriate for the proposed area of research.

Questions Reviewers May Ask about Supplies

✔ Are the major subcategories of supplies identified, such as animals, chemicals, and glassware?

✔ Where applicable, are unit prices shown?

✔ How has the rate of usage been determined?

Travel

Describe the purpose of the travel, the destination, and the individual(s) for whom the funds are requested. Remember, PHS policy requires that less than first-class air travel be used. Foreign travel must be justified in detail, describing its importance to the accomplishment of the project. And remember that a U.S. carrier must be used even if it causes increase in cost and/or inconvenience to the traveler.

Include cost of transportation for subjects and interviewers in the travel category, but calculate and indicate separately in the budget justification so that it is recognized as such. Make sure that your estimates conform to the guidelines of the awarding agency as well as your Institution.

Travel: Do Nots

✔ Do not ask to attend a scientific meeting that is clearly outside your area of research.

✔ Do not overstate mileage and per diem cost over federally approved maximum guidelines.

Questions Reviewers May Ask about Travel

✔ Is the amount of, and reason for, the anticipated travel consistent with the goals of the research project and with the amount of effort that the investigator will devote to the project?

✔ Has special justification been provided for any foreign travel requested?

Patient Care Costs

Provide the names of the hospitals to be used and the amounts requested for each, with an indication of the currently effective (DHHS) negotiated hospitalization rate agreement. If no rate agreement exists, indicate the basis that is used for calculating charges, including the number of patient days, estimated costs per day, and cost per test or treatment. Check your estimates with the hospital, and, for your protection, obtain a written quote. Make sure, as with the supplies connected with proposed tests, that the logic of the patient flow and your cost estimates coincide with the number of patients and dollars. Check to determine whether nursing care or technician's time are needed. Patient Care Costs do not include travel, per diem, or volunteer subject/donor fees. These costs should be requested in the "Other Expenses" category. Requests for consultant physician fees are to be reflected in the "Consultant Costs" category.

Patient Care Costs: Do Nots

- ✔ Do not request funds for coverage of laboratory tests that are routinely provided as part of a patient's basic tests.

Questions Reviewers May Ask about Patient Care Costs

- ✔ Are the proposed types and volume of tests necessary for the proposed research?
- ✔ Are the costs valid and reasonable in comparison with the expected results?

Alterations and Renovations

Requests for alterations and renovations (A&R) must be in accordance with permissible charges as allowed by the DHHS/PHS/NIMH. Indicate the purpose to be accomplished by the A&R, the location, the square footage involved, and the basis for the requested costs, such as an architect's or contractor's detailed cost estimate. The cost estimate should be dated with an indication as to how long the estimate is valid. When possible and where practicable, submit line drawings of the proposed renovations. Requests for costs of construction, per se, are not allowable. Your Institution must participate in estimating these costs and writing the detailed justification.

Other Expenses

This category may be used to itemize other expenses, such as publication costs, page charges, and books, by category and by unit cost. Reimbursement is allowable for tuition remission in lieu of all or part of salary for student work on the project. State on page 5 the percentage of tuition requested in proportion to the time devoted to the project. As mentioned earlier, this category may also be used for patient travel, per diem costs, and volunteer subject/donor fees.

Questions Reviewers May Ask about Other Expenses

- ✔ Have maintenance costs for laboratory animals been included?
- ✔ Have these costs been estimated on the basis of the guidelines for the care of laboratory animals?
- ✔ Does the project require purchased services from third parties or other institutions?
- ✔ If so, has the need for third-party indirect costs been anticipated?

Consortium/Contractual Costs

This category is intended to reflect the costs associated with the portion(s) of the requested research that is/are performed by an organization other than the proposed grantee. The participating or consortium

Institution is entitled to the same costs as the proposed grantee (e.g., personnel, supplies, equipment, travel, etc.) There is, however, a distinction to be made in the payment of indirect costs. The grantee Institution is paid indirect costs to cover its portion of the research, just as it is on any research grant without consortium activity.

On the other hand, the indirect costs for the third-party organization must be included in its requested budget, which therefore becomes a part of the grantee's direct-cost request. Indirect costs should be requested, applying the consortium organization's prevailing rate to the base that is represented in the proposed budget. The amount is to be reflected in the "Indirect Costs" line of the Consortium/Contractual Costs category of the detailed budget page for the third-party organization.

Separate budgets for the initial and future budget period must be prepared for each organization involved in consortium. The separate detailed budgets should clearly indicate a consortium arrangement. Use photocopies of pages 4 and 5 to itemize and justify budgets for the first 12-month period and for the entire proposed project period for each participating organization. The grantee's page 4 should then reflect the name of the consortium institution, the total costs (including indirect costs) requested for the third-party effort, and a reference to the attached separate detailed budget.

In some instances, contractual arrangements (purchase services) for major support services, such as laboratory testing of biological materials or clinical services, are of sufficient scope to warrant a similar categorical breakdown of costs, including indirect costs, if any. Be sure to show in item No. 9 of the face page the consortium organization's name, address, and EIN.

Questions Reviewers May Ask about Consortium/Contractual Costs

✔ Does the project require purchased services from third parties or other institutions?

✔ If so, has the need for third-party indirect costs been anticipated?

Other Support

Describe other support for each professional, including the PI, by time and effort:

✔ Active support

✔ Applications and proposals pending review or funding

Include a proposal for rearranging the priorities to ensure that the total time and effort does not exceed 100% for any of the listed personnel. Address in detail potential overlap in scientific content.

Noncompeting Continuation Applications

The noncompeting continuation application (Type 5) is generally limited to direct costs and may not exceed the recommended commitment included in the original competitive award. The budget is presented in a format similar to the competitive application and should generally be in line with the categorical recommendations developed during the competitive review; however, the grantee may exercise a reasonable degree of rebudgeting flexibility between and among the specific categories.

If institution-wide increases above those originally proposed and approved are to be considered by staff of the awarding component, full justification must be included in the application. Some examples of funding changes include: (1) cost of living adjustment of institution salaries; (2) fringe benefit rate increases; and (3) increases in the cost of supplies and services obtained from a central resource.

Be sure to illustrate clearly how the requested increase was determined. Remember that the increases can be calculated only on the "base" amount that generated the recommended level for the future year at the time that competing application was reviewed and approved. Inclusion of items outside the "base" represent expansion and cannot be considered administratively. Any favorable consideration will also be influenced by the availability of funds.

Finally, a few words about the flexibility that you may have once an award is made. In the United States there are institutional approaches to post-award administration. The largest universities participate in the Federal Demonstration Project. Most smaller Institutions are allowed to operate under the Expanded Authorities for Grantee Organizations, and the smallest ones have to go to the awarding Institution for all changes that they may require. Only certain types of grants qualify for this authority even within an Institution that participates in this program.

Federal Demonstration Project–Summary

- ✔ Relatedness–accountability for the project, not for the award
- ✔ Carryover of unobliged balance
- ✔ Elimination of most Prior Approvals
- ✔ Changes in grant period and pre-award costs

Expanded Authority for Grantee Organizations–Summary

- ✔ Extension without additional funds
- ✔ Pre-award costs
- ✔ Carryover of unobligated balances
- ✔ Cost-related Prior Approvals Authorities

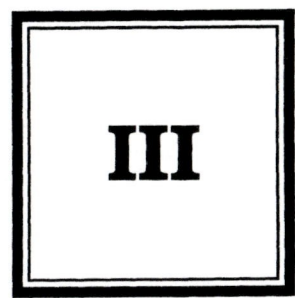

III

Disseminating Your Findings

Now that you have collected your data, you will want to make presentations to your colleagues and at scientific meetings. The following two chapters provide you with guidelines of how to prepare a better scientific talk that is enhanced by a well-prepared slide presentation. Janet B. W. Williams discusses both the process of developing the verbal content of your talk as well as its verbal presentation. Jeffrey Aarons and Robert Dunwoody develop points to be considered in designing the actual text to be used in your slides.

19

How to Deliver a Sensational Scientific Talk

Janet B. W. Williams

"Lectures were once necessary, but now when all can read, and books are numerous, lectures are unnecessary."

—Samuel Johnson

Samuel Johnson notwithstanding, talks are an indispensable part of professional life. This chapter provides guidelines on preparing and giving an effective presentation of a scientific paper. Readers will undoubtedly recall hearing many talks whose impacts were severely compromised by the lack of organization and ineffective style of presentation. Preparing a scientific paper for presentation is very different from writing a paper for publication; the public speaker must offer more to the audience than they can glean from reading a manuscript. The presentation must be entertaining, as well as cogent and well-paced, in order to get across to the audience a discussion of a study or topic in the most effective way.

The Initial Preparation: Thinking about the Talk

The title of your talk, publicized in the program, is the first exposure the audience has to you. It will influence how large your audience will be and how you will eventually be received, so it should be catchy yet informative. A glance through the program of any meeting, paying attention to the titles that "grab" you, should give you some ideas. A good title is well worth the amount of time devoted to its development.

Before pen is put to paper, the other important and useful work involves thinking about the audience. Typically, audiences at research meetings are mixed professionally. You should ask yourself how familiar they are likely to be with your topic, and, given that, what will be of most interest to them—not to you. The failure of many talks to hit home with an audience is due to the fact that the speaker did not gear the talk to the interests and background of that audience.

Once these points have been thought through, you can establish the scope of your talk by outlining the main ideas you want to cover. Initially these can be listed as broad statements, not necessarily in logical order. Once this list is completed, however, it is usually necessary to cut the number of ideas in half and limit yourself to only part of what you think might be included. The biggest mistake beginning public speakers make is to overload the talk with too many main ideas. Once the final list of ideas is developed, they should be put in a logical sequence for presentation.

As you work through this phase of preparation and the next, do not overestimate the audience's background or ability to absorb new ideas. When reading an article, the reader can take as much time as necessary to absorb new ideas, but, in a talk, if one crucial point is missed, the rest of the talk may not be understandable. It is far better to cover slowly and carefully a relatively small amount of material than to cover many points, however brilliantly, if half the audience gets lost.

Style of Delivery

To read or not to read? Your style of delivery is one of the most crucial factors determining how well your talk will be received. Most audiences prefer to listen to a spoken talk than one that is read in any form. When reading a paper the speaker keeps his or her eyes cast down and is not free to make gestures with the arms and hands, since they must be ready to turn pages. Contrast this style with one in which the speaker can make frequent eye contact with the audience, looking at each of the listeners one by one, and can make communicative facial expressions and body gestures to emphasize key points. Thus, the "speaker" (rather than the "reader") can use eyes, arms and hands, and torso as tools for effective communication, in addition to voice inflection. In addition, the speaker who is not tied to a sheaf of papers is free to move out from behind the podium to be in closer contact with the audience.

Because the speaker must be actively thinking through the ideas in order to present them coherently, there will be natural pauses (often sorely lacking in read presentations) between main ideas as both the audience and the speaker absorb the point and prepare for the next one. In normal speech our rate and inflection vary greatly, in contrast to reading, which tends to be steady in pace and monotonous in tone. In addition, spoken language differs in its sentence construction from written language, and it is easier for an audience to follow the generally shorter, more simply constructed and more emphatic sentences of spoken language. If one goal of public speaking is dramatic entertainment, then surely this technique is a requirement. The speaker does, however, have to remember to speak loudly enough to be heard in all parts of the room, and slowly (approximately 100–120 words per minute). The rate should be varied in order to avoid monotony, and the slowest pace should be during the parts of the talk with the most difficult content.

Despite audience preference, however, many presenters read their papers. The reasons for this seem obvious: When you are nervous, you are afraid you will not be able to concentrate on the content of your talk and present it in the most effective way. You think: "It's better to read the talk than to flub it." There are techniques you can use to organize your presentation so that you can talk from notes and still minimize the chances of disaster.

A fairly conservative strategy is to have your written paper in a notebook on the left-hand pages. On each right-hand page, then, outline corresponding notes of the points you would like to make. With this approach, you can feel confident speaking from the notes, knowing that if you panic the proper place in the written text is right there to fall back on. An alternative strategy, but perhaps a little riskier, involves writing out your speech, word for word, but then making notes from that text a few days before the presentation, and speaking from the notes at the final meeting. With this approach you can become thoroughly practiced in the exact phrasing you want to use, and for the actual talk you will have notes available as cues.

Table 1. Suggestions for Opening Attention-Getters

Tell a joke or show a cartoon. It is not absolutely necessary that the joke or cartoon be relevant to the topic, since any opener that gets the audience relaxed and engaged serves its purpose. If the joke can be related to the topic, however, so much the better; for example, begin with "You may think you've heard this talk before. . ." for a lecture on the *deja vu* phenomenon.

Begin with a bold, challenging statement: "There is no relationship between diagnosis and treatment."

Ask the DSM-IV audience a question. "How many of you have a copy of DSM-IV?" (Show of hands.) "How many of you have opened it?" (*Laughter*–fewer hands.)

Recount a personal experience. This can be related to your previous affiliation with the facility or meeting at which the talk is being given or a personal relationship with the person who introduced you.

Relate the lecture subject to a topical event. "A recent article in the *New York Times* described . . ."

Use a quote (as I did for this paper). This can be a quote from antiquity, for historical perspective on the topic, or a recent quotation. Whatever is chosen, it should introduce a controversial tone so that the audience looks forward to an interesting discussion.

State an informative but little-known fact that is of special relevance to the topic. (e.g., "In a well-known anxiety disorders clinic, social phobia is the third most common anxiety disorder.")

Relate your topic to a well-known research study or program. For example, in a talk on the cost of mental health care, you could begin with, "The Epidemiologic Catchment Area Program tells us that 30% of all Americans have had a mental disorder at some time in their lives."

Many lecturers find that the easiest and most effective way of using notes is to use slides to provide an outline for their talk. One or more slides can be presented for each main idea introduced, ensuring proper sequencing of the flow of the talk. This helps the audience follow along and allows the speaker to be less dependent on written notes.[1]

The Introduction

The way you begin your talk will be crucial for relaxing both your audience and you and for capturing their interest in your topic. Take the time to develop a powerful beginning; you should not be timid at this point. The introduction and conclusion of a talk, although they take the least time to give, take the most time to prepare.

Getting into the Talk

Following the introduction, the speaker should draw a "verbal map" for the audience of the sequence of the main points to follow. Then during the talk, at each major crossroad, the map should be reiterated. Each point should be clear to the audience before the next one is introduced. A speaker can assess if this is true by continually scanning the audience for puzzled looks or nods of heads.

[1] Editors' note: See "Developing a More Viewable Visual Presentation" by Aarons and Dunwoody, this volume.

In most cases, in which the purpose of a talk is to present the results of a study, the speaker should begin with the initial hypotheses and then present a description of the observations and a summary of the conclusions. Unlike a published paper, the method used should be described only briefly, with the talk concentrating instead on the results of the study. The audience can always ask questions about details of the method during the discussion period. See Table 1 for attention-getting openers.

Closing the Talk

A strong finish to your talk is nearly as important as a strong beginning. The ending is the climax and should be planned with care. You want the audience to know that you are changing pace, winding down the talk, and preparing for the discussion period. They should listen with a different kind of attention to your concluding statements.

To carry your closing words through to a strong finish, it is helpful to follow your final words with "Thank you." This gives the audience a clear signal that the talk is over, and it is time for them to clap. It avoids the uncomfortable situation that occurs when the speaker knows he or she has finished talking, but the audience thinks it is only a pause. Be sure to end on time so that there is adequate discussion time. (See also Table 2.)

The Discussion Period

Although the talk is over, you must remain alert for the discussion period. Prepare for the discussion period by trying to anticipate the most likely questions. Listen to the questions as they are being asked, nod approvingly to indicate you have understood them, and take notes if necessary. Never interrupt the questioner, even if you are certain you know what is being asked. Unless the question is asked from a microphone or can be very clearly heard, the audience will appreciate your repeating each question. This also ensures that you have understood it and gives you a bit more time to organize your response. When

---

Table 2. Different Strategies to Close a Talk

Change the tempo of delivery by slowing down your speech or pausing before you make your final comments.

Use signal words such as "finally" or "in conclusion," or refer to the audience as you move to your final statements. ("And so, as I've tried to show you . . .") This helps the audience keep in tune with the pace of the talk and prepare them to pay a different kind of attention to the ending.

Summarize what you have said, enumerating your conclusions. If you have been using slides, you should continue with a few phrases after the lights have been turned on.

Return to the opening statement. If your opener was a controversial fact or quote, you can now readdress it in light of the new information that you have presented.

Introduce a quotation that confirms your conclusions or sheds new light on the issue now that you have presented relevant data.

answering a question, pay tribute to it if it is deserved. ("That's a very interesting question . . .") This is also useful in disarming a questioner if the question is challenging or critical. If possible, reply with the questioner's name, and look at him or her as you answer.

In your replies, be brief and to the point, but not abrupt. If the answer to a question is lengthy and not of interest to the general audience, provide a brief response and invite the questioner to discuss it with you after the talk. If you simply do not know the answer to a particular question, do not be afraid to acknowledge ignorance. Such a disadvantage can sometimes be turned to an advantage by asking if anyone in the audience knows the answer to the question.

Practice, Practice, Practice

The most useful preparation for talk is practice. A good program of practice can be divided into three phases. Early practice, a few weeks before the talk is scheduled, should be done alone or with a significant other. Peace and quiet are essential for concentration. You should have a provisional outline or script of your talk and drafts of the slides (and other audiovisual aids) that you plan to use. You can use a tape recorder to listen to yourself and a clock to time the talk. The purpose of this early practice is to smooth out the outline of the talk and revise the audiovisual materials and to work on your grammar, the coordination of the verbal and visual components of the presentation, your timing and body gestures, and voice intonation. During this stage you should ensure that your talk fits within the necessary time limit. If you are using written text at this stage, it is helpful to know that one double-spaced written page takes about 1½ to 2 minutes to read.

At least two to three weeks prior to your presentation, you can begin intermediate practice. This can be a rehearsal with family, friends, or colleagues. Some academic departments require rehearsals within their own departments, each followed by critiques from the audience on the text, audiovisual aids, and manner of presentation. One must put one's ego aside during this stage and humbly accept criticism on any aspect of the talk, remembering that it is best to have deficiencies exposed by this small familiar group and have a chance to correct them before presenting to a large audience of relative strangers. The ability to accept and make use of such critiques is a true strength. At the end of this phase of practice, the slides should be finalized and sent off to the graphics designer.

One to two weeks before the talk, the final practice should take place, in private, concentrating on the introduction and conclusion to get them just right. Some find the shower a good place to practice, since it is both efficient and forces you to speak without even notes. The last week before the talk, if not before, the final speaking notes should be prepared.

Overcoming Nervousness

Even the most experienced speakers may be nervous at the beginning of a talk. Most find, however, that as they begin to focus on the content of the talk, much of their anxiety dissipates. Some degree of anxiety is adaptive in keeping you alert and in a state of readiness. However, some people have such a high level of anxiety that it interferes with their effectiveness as a public speaker.

It is important to realize that most speakers' anxiety is about the possibility of their nervousness being visible to the audience. A cycle takes over in which you are so afraid the audience will notice your nervousness that you become more anxious and afraid you will become immobilized and actually unable to continue the talk.

Two strategies may be helpful. First, it is worthwhile to remember that the statistical likelihood of your becoming totally incapacitated during the talk is much less than that of there being a total power failure during your talk. An informal mini-survey revealed that no one, despite years of attendance at professional meetings, could remember a single instance in which a speaker had to stop in the middle of a talk and could not continue. Secondly, you must realize that a speaker is always much more aware of his or her anxiety than others are. For this reason, many nervous speakers are amazed to hear comments after their talk about how good they were and how relaxed they seemed.

Conclusion

Public speaking can be a rewarding experience. It is a wonderful feeling to have delivered a talk successfully and to know that you have taught the audience something useful and meaningful. Taking my own advice, I will end with a quote that I hope this paper will help obviate:

> *"The scientific man [sic] is the only person who has anything new to say and who does not know how to say it."*
>
> —*Sir James Barrie*

20

Developing a More Viewable Visual Presentation

Jeffrey M. Aarons and Robert Dunwoody

Slides or videos can enhance a presentation by complementing and highlighting your message, but they can easily detract if they are unclear or too complex. The following are some of the steps that you can use to ensure better visual presentations.

Screening Situation

If possible, prior to developing your visual presentation, try to find out as much as possible about the room in which you will be making your presentation. The following information would be useful in designing your slide presentation:

✔ Room size

✔ Size of screen

✔ Distance to projector

✔ Distance from screen to back row

✔ Lighting

✔ Audience size

Due to time constraints, it is often difficult to plan slide compositions for a specific place (lecture hall, etc.). It is often more practical to create a standard format (e.g., a signature-graded or seamed-in background) for the routine bullet and chart slides and a variable background for other designs. This will allow you to combine sides for different presentations because they will blend together. For more sophisticated compositions all parameters may be altered.

You will not have control over many of the factors in the screening situation, so it is important to control the ones you do, which will be discussed below: (1) visual concepts, (2) amount of information, (3) size of type, and (4) use of color.

Visual Concepts

Generally it is better to show a progression of visual concepts that build up to a complex one rather than showing only the complex one for a longer period. By understanding the possibilities, we can effectively coordinate the content, relationship, and duration of sequential images presented in the form of slides. You can prepare your slides to develop an outline of your presentation that will help the audience understand the progression of your talk. See Table 1 for two different concept presentations.

The type of visual representation of your data can also be important. If you are trying to communicate change over time, either a line graph (Figure 1) or bar graph (Figure 2) can be effective. If, on the other hand, you are trying to communicate a comparison or proportion, a pie chart (Figure 3) or divided bars (Figure 4) may be better in communicating your message.

Table 1. Different Progression of Concepts in Slide Show

Title of Presentation	Title of Presentation
Research Team	Research Team
Point A	**Point A**
	Point B
	Point C
Point A-1	Point A-1
Point A-2	Point A-2
Point A-3	Point A-3
Point A	Point A
Point B	**Point B**
	Point C
Point B-1	Point B-1
Point B-2	Point B-2
Point B-3	Point B-3
Point A	Point A
Point B	Point B
Point C	**Point C**
Point C-1	Point C-1
Point C-2	Point C-2
Point C-3	Point C-3
Point A	Point A
Point B	Point B
Point C	Point C
Conclusion	Conclusion

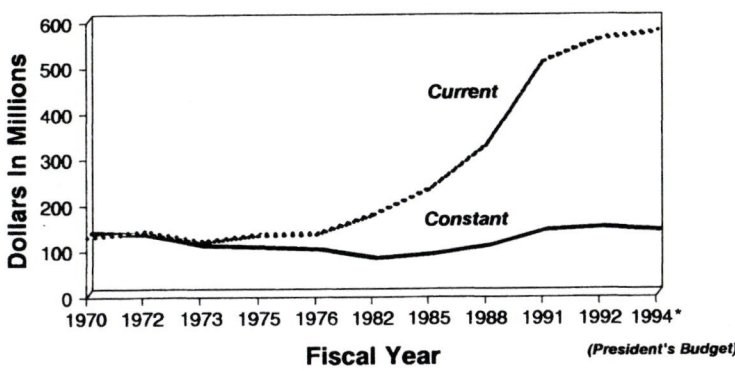

Figure 1. Example of a line graph.

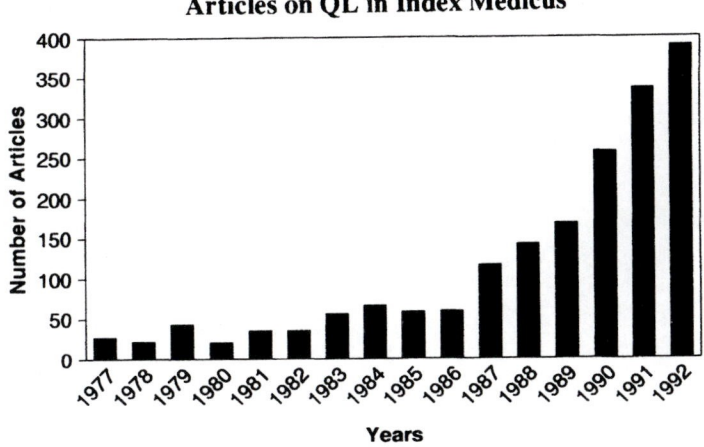

Figure 2. Example of a bar graph.

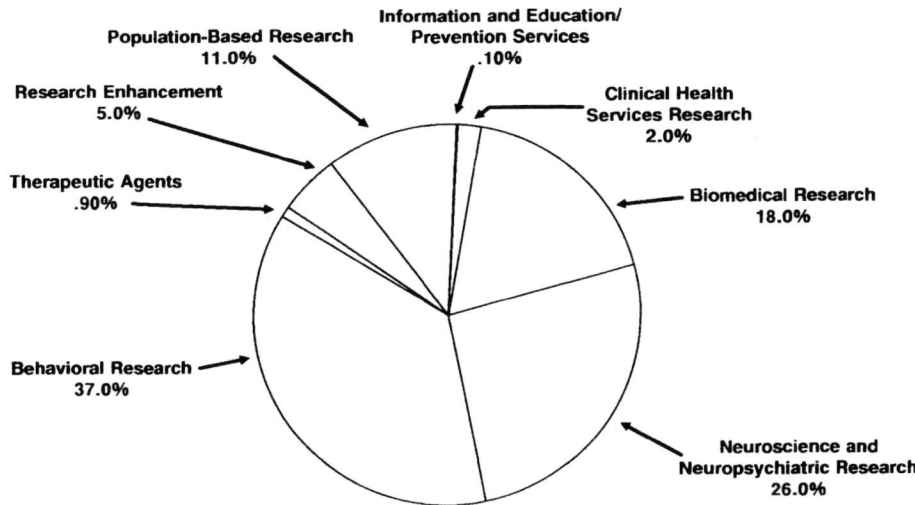

Figure 3. Example of a pie graph.

**Reported Cases of AIDS and
Case-Fatality Rates by Half Year of
Diagnosis, United States**

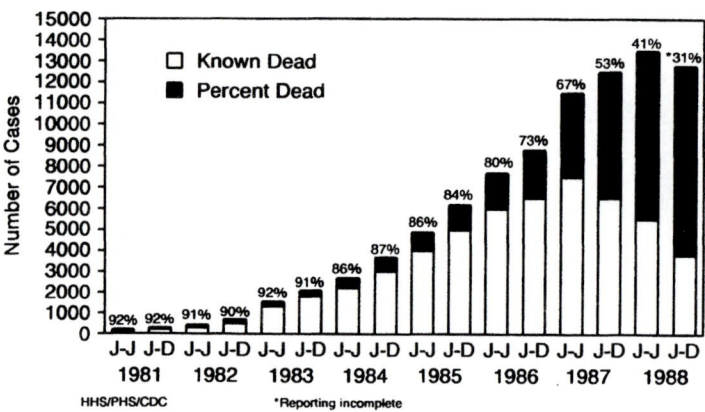

Figure 4. Example of a divided bar graph.

Amount of Information

Depending on whether the target audience is an educated lay audience or experts in the subject matter, you should match the visual elements and content to their level. The subject matter and its inherent complexity often determine whether the information can be clearly presented as one slide or as a sequence of slides or video images, resulting in a form of rudimentary animation.

Table 2. Using Phrases rather than Sentences

Sentences: Consensus on interventions (poor example)

The consensus of NIMH grantees on designing intervention: (1) AIDS prevention programs are more successful if they are integrated into ongoing systems of care (e.g., STD clinic, family medicine clinics, etc.); (2) prevention strategies should be tailored to the specific population, should involve participation by the community, and should be led by persons with whom the participants can identify; and (3) in the hierarchy of concerns of persons at risk for HIV infection, housing, crime, and unemployment may rank higher than HIV risk and need to be addressed prior to implementing HIV prevention programs.

Phrases: Consensus on interventions (good example)

Integrated into ongoing systems of care

Prevention strategies should be:
   community participation
   tailored to population
   peer-led groups

Housing, crime, unemployment of greater concern than AIDS

Table 3. Presenting Statistical Data (Poor Example).
HIV-Related Behavior of Women Prior to Intervention[a]

Variable	Treatment Group (n = 100)		Standard Care Group (n = 50)	
	M	SD	M	SD
Age	21	3	23	5
Years of education	10	2	12	3
Household income	2	2	4	2
Number of children	3	1	2	2
Assertiveness scale score	3.5	0.8	3.7	.5
Number reporting unprotected sex	3.8	3	2.3	3
Total number of lifetime sexual partners	14	8	16	9
Total number of partners in last 30 days	3	1	2	1
Total number of partners in last week	1	2	1	1
Percentage reporting condom use	7		4	
Percentage reporting chlamydia	8		10	
Percentage reporting gonorrhea	11		12	
Percentage reporting alcohol use	44		22	
Percentage reporting drug use	38		27	
Percentage reporting sex for drugs	25		17	
Percentage with condoms at interview	12		8	
AIDS knowledge of test score	25.3	3.3	26.3	20
Anxiety score	37.1	9	40	3
Depression score	6.8	5.5	8.9	12.1
Internal locus of control score	15.1	4.6	15.7	10
				3.7

[a] This data is not real but is presented to make a point.

Table 4. Presenting Statistical Data (Good Example).
HIV-Related Behavior of Women Prior to Intervention

Variable	Treatment Group (n = 100)		Standard Care Group (n = 50)	
	M	SD	M	SD
Age	21	3	23	5
Years of education	10	2	12	3
Number of children	3	1	2	2
Assertiveness scale score	3.5	0.8	3.7	0.5
Total number of partners in last 30 days	3	1	2	1
Percentage reporting condom use	7		4	
Percentage reporting STDs	20		12	
AIDS knowledge of test score	25.3	3.3	26.3	3

Ordinarily you should use the slide to highlight your critical points and you should not read it. If you quote someone verbatim on a slide, let the audience read it while you discuss the concept more generally.

Edit material carefully to keep it simple, and present phrases rather than sentences. You should edit down to key words or statements so that the audience can understand your major points. Table 2 presents an example of how much more effective well-chosen phrases are than sentences.

When presenting statistical data you should keep it simple and focused. Often, the speaker will quickly flash a complicated table with multiple columns and rows with the lame comment that this supports his or her point. More potent support for the point might have been made better by a simplified table directing the viewer to the specific point that is being made. Table 3 presents an example of statistics being presented that is too complex for an oral presentation but would be appropriate for a journal article. Table 4 provides a manageable amount of data for one slide.

Size of Type

Formulas are available to calculate text size on slides as a function of room size, but there is an easy pre-projection test. If you can you read the text or see all the detail in the graphic image when you simply hold the slide in front of you at arm's length without any magnification, then it probably will be readable.

If possible, you should design your slide for the last row of your audience and test the effectiveness of the size of type selected prior to your presentation. Remember, there is an inverse relationship between the number of words and/or numbers on a slide and size of the type size that you will be able to use.

Consult the graphic or computer artist for the appropriate type size. If you are using your own software (Harvard Graphics), for example, use type as large as possible with enough data to illustrate your points. Titles should be larger than text (7–10 points approximately). Titles should also be a different weight; bold should be used for titles, and medium weight should be used for text. Underlines can be effectively used to separate the title from the text. Subtitles should be about 3 points smaller than the title.

Use of Color

There are various computer-based and commercially available techniques for producing effective slides. Those with light-colored images on a dark background are the best ones for projecting in rooms that are not completely darkened. Backgrounds should be blue or black. Blue is more pleasing to the eye, and it also can be graded.

The most annoying characteristic of some slide and overhead transparency presentations at scientific meetings is poor contrast ratios. When combined with overly detailed content, this is frustrating to the audience. Titles should be different colors to stand out from the text. If you use white or yellow text on a black or blue background, you will bring attention to your text. Primary information such as major topics, specific data, and column of interest, should be highlighted with a different color. Consistent application of highlighting elements within a slide, such as bullets, lines, or graph data, will direct the attention of the audience to critical areas and prevent boredom.

The presenter should consult the graphic artist on the basic design structure, type font, and weights and colors used to establish a hierarchical order.

Number of Slides in Presentation

The number of slides selected for a talk will vary depending on the amount of information on the slide and the complexity of your presentation. A rule of thumb may be approximately 1–3 minutes per slide. Using this general principal, if you have ½ hour and all of your slides are complex, you should plan on approximately 10 slides. If the slides are simple, you might effectively use 25 slides.

Future Technology

Computer video animation is a format that is being developed and will be increasingly used in the future. This will allow you to provide even better visual illustrations for your talks (e.g., PET scans, neuropsychological test administration, mock counseling sessions, etc.) but may initially require more effort on your part to develop a video that can be well integrated into your talk.

Conclusion

If you want to entertain, inform, and challenge people with your presentations, illustrate your ideas and other information with well-composed and exposed slides presented in a well-paced manner.

Information on the Authors

Jeffrey M. Aarons   Mr. Aarons has been a professional artist for over 20 years. He has worked as a medical illustrator at NIMH since 1983. Since 1987 he has been interested in enhancing the computer graphics capability of the Institute. He also creates a broad range of slides, which include everything from routine charts and graphs to sophisticated design elements and full-color medical anatomical illustrations, both clinical and conceptual. His illustrations have appeared in over 100 magazines, books, and journals over the years and on network television programs that featured prominent NIMH scientists.

Peter Adler, Ph.D.   Peter Adler is Professor of Sociology at the University of Denver, where he served as Chair from 1987–1993. Dr. Adler served as the editor of *Journal of Contemporary Ethnography* (1986–1994), as well as the founding editor of *Sociological Studies of Child Development* (1985–1992). He has authored and edited several books, including *Momentum, The Social Dynamics of Financial Markets, Membership Roles in Field Research, Backboards and Blackboards, and Constructions of Deviance*. His research interests include qualitative methodology, deviant behavior, and social psychology.

Hortensia Amaro, Ph.D.   Dr. Amaro is Professor of Social and Behavioral Sciences in the School of Public Health at Boston University. She has served as a consultant and in various advisory roles to the Surgeon General's Agenda on Hispanic Health, the Centers for Disease Control, the National Institutes of Health, the National Institute on Drug Abuse, and the Center for Substance Abuse Prevention, as well as with foundations and community-based organizations. She is founder and past president of the Latino Health Institute of Massachusetts and founder of the Multicultural AIDS Coalition and the National Hispanic Psychological Association. Dr. Amaro's research has focused on epidemiological studies and community-based interventions for substance abuse and HIV among women and on Hispanic health issues.

Robyn Dawes, Ph.D.   Dr. Dawes moved to Carnegie Mellon University in the fall of 1985, as a Professor of Psychology in the Department of Social and Decision Sciences and the department's head for a 5-year period. He has authored over 100 journal articles and 3 books (the latest, *Rational Choice in an Uncertain World*, 1986, Harcourt, Brace, Jovanovich). He also served for over 3 years on the National Research Council's Committee on AIDS Research and the Behavioral, Social Statistical Sciences and has contributed to its two reports: "AIDS, Sexual Behavior, and Intravenous Drug Use" (1989), and

"AIDS: The Second Decade" (1990). He served as a member of the AIDS Review Committee at NIMH.

Robert Dunwoody   Mr. Dunwoody received a Master of Fine Arts degree in 1985 from American University, then took a six-month painting sabbatical. After this, he returned to work, pursuing a career in illustration with the U.S. Federal Government. From there he transferred to the Defense Mapping Agency (DMA) in a graphics designer position and learned computer graphics and video production. Mr. Dunwoody later transferred from DMA to NIMH to further pursue career opportunities in video production and computer graphics and is at present a computer graphics artist with the Technical Services Branch, Office of Scientific Information.

Eleanor Friedenberg, R.N., M.S.   Ms. Friedenberg, R.N., M.S., has been the Director of the Division of Extramural Activities (DEA) for the National Institute for Drug Abuse (NIDA) since 1992. Prior to her DEA assignment, Ms. Friedenberg was Deputy Director, Division of Prevention and Special Mental Health Programs, which managed the research activities of several Centers, including the Center for Minority Mental Health Studies. Ms. Friedenberg holds a master's degree in psychiatric nursing and began at NIMH in 1961.

Richard B. Fritz, Ph.D.   Dr. Fritz earned his Ph.D. in sociology from Northwestern University in Evanston, Illinois. He is currently Associate Professor of Sociology at Saint Xavier University in Chicago, where he is conducting research on the relationship between coping resources, AIDS knowledge, and condom usage among high-risk women. From 1989–1992, Dr. Fritz served as Research Director for the Comprehensive AIDS Prevention and Education Program, jointly sponsored by the Centers for Disease Control and the Chicago Department of Health, which evaluated community-based AIDS prevention programs for female street prostitutes, runaway teens, gay and lesbian youth, and jail inmates. His work includes "Computer Analysis of Qualitative Data," in NIDA Research Monograph 98: *The Collection and Interpretation of Data From Hidden Populations,* and "How Effective Are AIDS Prevention Programs for High-Risk Populations: An Evaluation of Four AIDS Education Programs in Chicago," which was presented at the VIII International Conference on AIDS.

Paul Goldstein, Ph.D.   Dr. Goldstein is currently an Associated Professor in the School of Public Health, University of Illinois, Chicago. He is the author of several books, as well as numerous articles and chapters. His research into the connections between drugs and violence has been supported by both the National Institute on Drug Abuse and the National Institute of Justice. Dr. Goldstein's current research interests include patterns and consequences of anabolic–androgenic steroid use and a wide variety of issues associated with the nexus between violence and families, including substance use, marital violence, child abuse, and pregnancy.

Gregory Herek, Ph.D.   Dr. Herek is currently an Associate Research Psychologist in the Department of Psychology, AIDS Psychosocial Research Group, University of California at Davis. Dr. Herek's research interests focus on using social psychological research on attitudes, persuasion, and communication to improve AIDS public education programs and to reduce AIDS-related stigma. He currently is funded by NIMH for two projects: (1) an application of social psychological theory and research to AIDS educational videos and (2) a national survey study of Americans' reactions to the AIDS epidemic. In addition to his work on AIDS, Dr. Herek has published extensively on the topics of anti-gay violence and prejudice.

Jeffrey Kelly, Ph.D.   Dr. Kelly is presently Director of the NIMH-funded Center for AIDS Intervention Research (CAIR) and Professor of Psychiatry and Mental Health Sciences at the Medical College of Wisconsin in Milwaukee. Dr. Kelly's research focuses on the application of behavior change principles to

HIV risk reduction as well as mental health aspect of AIDS/HIV. Dr. Kelly is the author of approximately 150 articles, book chapters, and books, primarily addressing HIV prevention and mental health issues. He has served on the editorial boards of numerous psychology journals and is presently an Associate Editor of *Health Psychology.*

Janice Kiecolt-Glaser, Ph.D. Dr. Kiecolt-Glaser has been on the faculty in the Department of Psychiatry in The Ohio State University College of Medicine since 1978, and she currently holds the rank of professor. In collaboration with Dr. Ronald Glaser, Professor and Chair of Medical Microbiology and Immunology, she codirects a large interdisciplinary research and training program addressing psychological influences on immunity. Their work together began in 1982 and has focused on such diverse groups as medical students, newlywed couples, and family members who are caregiving for an Alzheimer's disease victim.

Thomas R. N. Lalley, M.A. Dr. Lalley is Chief, Services Research Branch, National Institute of Mental Health. In this capacity, he oversees a multidisciplinary research and research grant program that covers the fields of mental health services research and mental health economics, with special attention to mental health services for persons with severe mental illness, children and adolescents, and minority populations. Prior to assuming his current post, Mr. Lalley served as Deputy Chief of the NIMH Antisocial and Violent Behavior Branch.

Barry Lebowitz, Ph.D. Dr. Lebowitz is Chief of the Mental Disorders of the Aging Research Branch of the National Institute of Mental Health and a member of the adjunct faculty of the Department of Psychiatry of the Georgetown University School of Medicine. A frequent participant in public and scientific forums, Dr. Lebowitz serves on the editorial boards of a number of professional scientific journals and has made many published contributions to the literature of gerontology and geriatrics.

Raymond P. Lorion, Ph.D. Dr. Lorion is on the faculty at the University of Maryland at College Park. Since 1984, he has served as Senior Policy consultant to the Office of the Administrator of ADAMHA, to the White House Office of Drug Abuse Policy, and to various state and local agencies regarding the development and evaluation of prevention programs. Dr. Lorion has written or edited ten books and 60 chapters and scientific papers. The majority of his publications focus on the design, evaluation, and implementation of community-based preventive interventions targeted to responding to the needs of children at risk for emotional and behavioral disorders. He is currently working on a long-term epidemiological study of factors associated with the onset, maintenance, and cessation of alcohol and drug use in children.

William Lyman, Ph.D. Dr. Lyman is currently an Associate Professor of Pathology and Neuroscience in both departments at Albert Einstein College of Medicine. Dr. Lyman has won a number of national awards for his research in the areas of autoimmune disease and AIDS. He has served as a member on a number of national advisory committees and is currently a member of the NIMH AIDS Study Section. He has been a grant awardee from the National Institute of Mental Health and has also received both program project grants and R01s from NINDS and NIDA.

Spero M. Manson, Ph.D. A Pembina Chippewa of the Turtle Mountain Reservation, Dr. Manson, since 1986, has been a Professor, Department of Psychiatry, University of Colorado Health Sciences Center, and Director, National Center for American Indian and Alaska Native Mental Health research, which is located at the same institution. Dr. Manson has served on numerous boards of directors.

Ali Manwar, Ph.D. Dr. Manwar was a National Institute on Drug Abuse Postdoctoral Fellow in Drug Abuse Research (1990–1993) at National Development and Research Institutes, Inc. (NDRI), New York. Later he joined NDRI on the project titled "The Natural History of Crack Distribution/Abuse." He has been awarded a Scientist Development Award (K21) from NIH/NIDA to study the household economics of the drug dealers. Previously, he received a Fulbright–Hays fellowship to conduct field research for his dissertation.

Leonard Mitnick, Ph.D. Dr. Mitnick is currently the Associated Director for Research Training in the Office on AIDS, NIMH. Between 1986 and 1992, Dr. Mitnick served as the Chief of the Basic Prevention and Behavioral Medicine Research Branch and its predecessor Division of Basic Brain and Behavioral Sciences, NIMH. Other experiences include research, teaching, and consulting.

Frank Mucha, M.B.A. Mr. Mucha has worked at Columbia University since 1969 in many areas connected with administration, accounting, private practice, grant management, and overall management, and is currently in Department of Psychiatry (1981 to present). He has developed an integrated (spread sheet–based) system for large program project/center grant applications enabling multi-institutional collaboration and its centralized administration. He has also participated in Initial Review Process, evaluation of administrative strengths and weaknesses of centers and programs.

Bryan Page, Ph.D. Dr. Page has participated in a wide variety of transdisciplinary studies, most of which required him to blend qualitative analytical skills with quantitative analysis. He has elicited and analyzed life and drug use histories of Costa Rican marijuana users in a study of that drug's long-term effects. Cuban polydrug users recruited in Miami's Little Havana neighborhood provided qualitative and quantitative data for his study of how some Cubans adapted to exile through drug use. Dr. Page also has studied prescription drug use among women, polydrug use among the Seminole Tribe of Florida, and alcohol use among Veterans Administration inpatients. His most recent research, funded by NIMH, involves HIV risk among Haitian women and multiple retroviral infection among intravenous drug users, with substantial qualitative components in each study.

Delores L. Parron, Ph.D. Dr. Parron is the Associate Director for Special Populations at the National Institute of Mental Health at the National Institutes of Health. She is co-editor (with David A. Hamburg and Glen R. Elliot) of *Health and Behavior, Frontiers of Research in the Biobehavioral Sciences,* and (with Frederic Solomon) *Mental Health Services in Primary Care Settings.*

Willo Pequegnat, Ph.D. Dr. Pequegnat is the Associate Director for Behavioral and Neuroscience Research in the Office on AIDS at the National Institute of Mental Health (NIMH). She serves as a specialist in neurobehavioral, psychosocial, and AIDS prevention research and has responsibility to plan, direct, and evaluate a national grant and contract program in several major interrelated research areas, including evaluation of existing and new neuropsychological, psychiatric, and neurological research programs for adult and pediatric HIV infection and AIDS; studies of the etiology and pathogenesis of the disease in special populations (e.g., women, adolescents, and children); and studies to develop new initiatives in AIDS prevention research.

Judith Godwin Rabkin, M.P.H., Ph.D. Dr. Rabkin has been a research scientist at New York State Psychiatric Institute for 20 years and is currently a Professor of Clinical Psychology at College of Physicians and Surgeons, Columbia University. She has been consecutively vice-chairman, co-chairman, and chairman of the IRB at New York State Psychiatric Institute, since 1979 and on occasion serves as a consultant to other IRBs in New York State. Dr. Rabkin has been engaged in AIDS research since 1987 as a co-investigator in the HIV center for Clinical and Behavioral Studies at Columbia, and is herself a grant recipient from NIMH in AIDS-related research. Finally, she was a member of the NIMH AIDS grant review committee. Accordingly, she has seen grants from all angles: as an applicant, as part of the IRB regulatory procedure, and as a grant reviewer.

Juan Ramos, Ph.D. Dr. Ramos has been at the National Institute of Mental Health since May 1968 and has held several positions since then, most significantly his twelve years as Director of the Division of Prevention and Special Mental Health Programs. Since 1985 he has been the Deputy Director for Prevention and Special Projects, with responsibility for certain aspects of AIDS, prevention, refugee mental health, international activities, and work related to Healthy People 2000 and, most recently, a Task Force on Social Work Research. During this period he has had a continuing interest in minority mental health concerns, especially those related to the Hispanic community, the development of social work research infrastructure, and prevention policy.

Robert Remien, Ph.D.　　Dr. Remien is conducting research full time at the HIV Center for Clinical and Behavioral Studies at the New York State Psychiatric Institute and Columbia University and is on the faculty in the Department of Psychiatry at Columbia University. He has been conducting research and publishing primarily in the area of psychiatric and psychosocial issues related to HIV infection. He is currently working on projects exploring alcohol and drug use behavior in the context of HIV and quality of life in a group of "long-term" survivors with AIDS. He also has a private clinical practice and continues to run a PWA therapy group as a volunteer at the Gay Men's Health Crisis in New York City.

Sherry Roberts　　Ms. Roberts began her career at the National Institute of Mental Health in 1980. During her tenure at the Institute, she has held numerous positions. She is currently a Program Specialist and Special Assistant to the Director, Office on AIDS. She participates with the Director in coordinating the planning, analysis, reporting, and management activities of the office. She is the office representative for administrative, budget, grant, and contract matters.

Hugh Stamper, Ph.D.　　Dr. Hugh Stamper began his NIH career as a program officer in the National Heart, Lung, and Blood Institute. He subsequently moved to the Division of Research Grants, where he served first as an executive secretary and then as a section chief. Since 1989, he has been Director, Division of Extramural Activities, National Institute of Mental Health. In this capacity he oversees the peer review of all grant applications that are assigned to the Institute at both the Initial Review Group and the National Advisory Mental Health Council level. He is also responsible for the development, oversight, and implementation within the Institute of policies regarding extramural grants and contracts.

Ellen Stover, Ph.D.　　Dr. Stover has served as the Director of the NIMH Office on AIDS since its establishment in 1988. She has been involved in guiding developments in the field of HIV research toward the development of strategies to reduce transmission of HIV and prevention of high-risk behaviors since 1983. Beginning in 1983 with a budget of $200,000, she has built the program into a $90-million program in 1995. Her efforts have led to the development of interdisciplinary AIDS research centers, a multisite, multipopulation study of behavioral approaches to prevent the spread of HIV, a Phase II clinical trial of an AIDS therapeutic, and efforts in the area of secondary prevention related to AIDS dementia.

Anselm Strauss, Ph.D.　　Dr. Strauss is Professor Emeritus of Sociology, Department of Social and Behavioral Sciences, University of California, San Francisco. His main research activities have been in the sociology of health and illness and in the sociology of work and professions. The research methods used in his studies have principally been a combination of field observation and interviews, but occasionally historical materials are used as primary data. Among his (and co-authors') books on method or monographs are: *The Discovery of Ground Theory* (1967), *Qualitative Analysis for Social Scientists* (1987), *Awareness of Dying* (1965), *The Social Organization of Medical Work* (1985), and *Unending Work and Care* (1988). He has been a visiting professor at the Universities of Cambridge, Paris, Manchester, Constance, Adelaide, and Hagen. His current research includes studies of AIDS policymaking and implementation, the flow of work in hospitals, and the role of the body in action.

Jose Szapocznik, Ph.D.　　Dr. Szapocznik, a clinical psychologist, is research Professor of Psychiatry, Director of the Spanish Family Guidance Center, Deputy Director of the Center for the Biopsychosocial

Study of AIDS, and Director of the Miami World Health Organization Collaborating Center for Research and Training in Mental Health, Alcohol, and Drug Dependence, all in the Department of Psychiatry at the University of Miami. Dr. Szapocznik is currently the only behavioral scientist in the congressionally mandated aids program advisory committee with the responsibility for providing guidance to the Secretary of Health, the Assistant Secretary of Health, and the Director of the National Institutes of Health on Aids Research Policy and Programs. He is a former consultant to numerous national (NIMH, NIDA, OSAP, ADAMHA, AOA, ORR, Headstart, etc.) and international (WHO, PAHO, United Nations) organizations, has nearly 100 publications, including a recent book, *Breakthroughs in Family Therapy with Drug Abusing and Problem Youth*, reporting on his original research. Dr. Szapocznik has distinguished himself for his theoretical, clinical, and research innovations in the field of family therapy and, in particular, in the family treatment of Hispanic drug using adolescents. He has also worked extensively and conducted research with ethnic minorities and on institutional racism.

H. Gerry Taylor, Ph.D. Dr. Taylor, has published papers and has been on national review boards in the fields of child development and behavioral medicine. He has also served as the Principal Investigator of multicenter study of the developmental consequences of meningitis and Director of McGill-Montreal Children's Hospital Learning Centre. He returned to the United States from Canada last year to become director of pediatric psychology at Rainbow Babies and Children's Hospital and to pursue his interests in learning disabilities and recovery of function following early brain insults.

Janet B. W. Williams, D.W.S. Dr. Williams is currently Professor of Clinical Psychiatric Social Work in the Departments of Psychiatry and Neurology at the College of Physicians and Surgeons, Columbia University, and a Research Scientist at the New York State Psychiatric Institute, where she is also Co-Director of the Biometrics Research Department. She is well-known for her work in research methodology and the assessment of psychopathology and for her involvement in the development of DSM-III, DSM-III-R, and DSM-IV.

Steven Zalcman, M.D. Dr. Zalcman is currently Chief of the Neuroimaging and Applied Neuroscience Research Branch in NIMH's Division of Basic Brain and Behavioral Sciences. Programs for which he has direct responsibility include the Neuroscience Centers Program, the Neuroimaging Program, and the Neural Systems Program. Dr. Zalcman is also playing a major role in NIMH's efforts to implement the Human Brain Project as a major activity in the Decade of the Brain.

Appendix A
Data Analytic Plan[1]

BB   PRINCIPAL INVESTIGATOR/PROGRAM DiRECTOR: <u>Karen Olness</u>

DESCRIPTION: State the application's broad, long-term objectives and specific aims, making reference to the health relatedness of the project. Describe concisely the experimental design and methods for achieving these goals. Avoid summaries of past accomplishments and the use of the first person. This abstract is meant to serve as a succinct and accurate description of the proposed work when separated from the application. **DO NOT EXCEED THE SPACE PROVIDED.**

This study proposes to examine the neurodevelopmental effects of HIV infection in a large and stable population of infants in Uganda. It will extend a follow-up study of HIV positive newborns that is ongoing in Uganda. We will assess the cognitive, development, and neurologic status from birth to 24 months of 320 Ugandan infants who are HIV positive at birth and 100 infants who are HIV negative at birth. Specific aims are (1) a prospective assessment of the neurodevelopmental consequences of HIV infection (birth to 24 months) using measures of cognitive development (Bayley Scale and Fagan Test of Infant Intelligence), language development, neurologic status, and behavior; (2) identification of the factors which predict cognitive and neurologic deterioration in HIV infected infants; (3) detailed assessment of potential covarying influences including maternal health, family environment, and child nutrition status. The following propositions will be examined: (1) HIV infection will be associated with deterioration in neurodevelopmental status that is not accounted for by covarying factors; (2) Children's visual recognition performance at three months of age will predict subsequent developmental and neurologic status. Neurologic exam and the Bayley Scale will be given at three month intervals for the first 12 months and repeated at 18 and 24 months. Home visits to study subjects will be made every two weeks for the first six months of life and monthly, thereafter, until age two. The proposed study will enhance knowledge of the neurodevelopmental consequences of HIV infection in infants and young children, generate new information concerning factors that influence cognitive and neurologic outcomes, and test the utility of visual recognition performance for early detection of cognitive and neurologic deterioration in HIV infected infants.

KEY PERSONNEL ENGAGED ON PROJECT

NAME, DEGREE(S), SSN	POSITION TITLE AND ROLE IN PROJECT	DEPARTMENT AND ORGANIZATION
K. Olness, M.D. #477-38-2520	Professor, Principal Invest.	Pediatrics Case Western Reserve Univ.
H. Hall, Ph.D., #292-52-2391	Asst. Prof., Co-PI	Pediatrics, CWRU
M. Wiznitzer, M.D. #331-44-4521	Asst. Prof., Co-PI	Pediatrics, CWRU
D. Drotar, Ph.D., #146-36-2389	Prof. of Psych. Co-PI	Psychiatry, CWRU
D. Hom, Ph.D., #283-42-6646	Asst. Prof. Co-PI	Epidemiology, CWRU
C. Ndugwa	Professor, Project Leader	Pediatrics Makerere University, Uganda
F. Mmiro	Professor, Project Leader	Obstetrics Makerere University, Uganda

A.   Specific Aims and Hypotheses

The increasing numbers of infants that are affected by HIV infection necessitate a more complete scientific understanding of the neurodevelopmental consequences of this condition. Conclusions that can be drawn from prior studies of the neurodevelopment of HIV infected infants and young children have been limited by salient methodological problems, especially small sample sizes, short follow-up periods, and failure to provide a comprehensive neurodevelopmental assessment or evaluate the impact of environmental influences. Designed to address these gaps in our understanding of the neurodevelopmental consequences of HIV infection, this prospective study will assess the cognitive development and neurological status from birth to 24 months of 320 Ugandan infants who are HIV positive at birth and 100 Ugandan infants who are HIV negative at birth. The proposed research will extend an ongoing, follow-up study of the infants of mothers who are HIV positive which is already organized and well in place.

The proposed study has the following specific aims: (1) assessment of the neurodevelopmental consequences of HIV infection in a prospective, controlled study using a comprehensive assessment of cognitive development (Bayley Scale and Fagan Test of Infant Intelligence), language, and neurological status, (2) identification of the factors that predict developmental and neurological deterioration in HIV infected infants; (3) detailed assessment of potential covarying influences on cognitive development such as children's nutritional status, maternal health and neurological status, and family demographics and caretaking.

The following hypotheses will be tested: 1) Infants with HIV infection will demonstrate neurodevelopmental deterioration not accounted for by covarying factors in comparison to controls without HIV infection. 2) Infants born HIV positive who are uninfected 15 months post-partum will demonstrate no greater neurodevelopmental deterioration than will control infants born HIV negative and uninfected at 15 months. 3) Visual recognition ability scores in infants born HIV positive who later demonstrate HIV infection will be lower than in control infants who are not infected with HIV.

We anticipate that findings from the proposed study will enhance knowledge of the neurodevelopmental consequences of HIV infection in infants and young children in several important ways. The prospective assessment of a cohort of HIV positive infants compared to a cohort of HIV negative infants will provide data concerning the course of cognitive development and neurological status associated with HIV infection. The proposed study will generate new information concerning factors that influence individual differences in the neurologic performance and developmental prognosis of HIV infected infants. Infant visual recognition memory performance might predict subsequent cognitive and neurologic deterioration.

B.   Background and Significance

Epidemiologic data indicate that the prevalence of HIV infection in infants in the U.S.A. and in the world is increasing dramatically (1). In Uganda the earliest cases of clinical AIDS were recognized in 1982 in Rakai district, in the southwestern part of the country. By the end of 1988, a cumulative total of about 6,500 AIDS cases had been reported to the Ministry of Health, including approximately 700 cases of AIDS in children under five years of age. It is likely that these figures are underestimates. Available data based on two or more screening tests using the Cambridge ELISA method to test pregnant Ugandan mothers in the Kampala area and their infants indicates that approximately 24% of these women are HIV positive. Clinical diagnoses of AIDS, based on WHO criteria, of hospitalized women and children at New Mulago Hospital of Makerere University are consistent with the high percentage of HIV serum positivity noted. In 1987, 42 percent of 1,328 in- and out-patients in 15 Ugandan hospitals had ELISA tests positive for HIV antibody.(2).

At the present time, there is little certainty about the vertical transmission rate in children born to HIV seropositive mothers. Reported rates have varied greatly from 12% to 73% (3, 4, 5). An unpublished study of 87 Ugandan infants born to HIV seropositive mothers in Kampala found that 19 (22%) of these children were infected as demonstrated by positive western blot results in children after age 15 months.

The large numbers of HIV infected infants necessitates more complete scientific understanding of the clinical manifestations and progression of the disease. HIV infection is a multi-faceted problem which is associated with a range of medical and psychological problems in children and affected families (1). Neurologic and cognitive impairments are among the most tragic and least understood clinical manifestations of HIV infection in affected adults and children. Adult patients in the later stages of HIV infection have been observed to suffer from a neurological syndrome characterized by abnormalities in cognition, motor performance, and behavior, known as AIDS dementia complex (2). Abnormalities in complex sequencing, fine and rapid motor movement, and neuropsychologic abnormalities have also been observed to be the sole manifestations of HIV infections in asymptomatic seropositive individuals (6-8).

Central nervous system impairments associated with HIV infection are not limited by age. In their comprehensive review of the clinical manifestation of human immunodeficiency in children, Faloon, et al (9) noted several reports of developmental delays, deterioration of motor skills and intellectual abilities and behavioral abnormalities characteristic of children with HIV infection. Intellectual deterioration in children with AIDS may be accompanied by paresis, pyramidal tract signs, ataxia, abnormal muscle tone or pseudobulbar palsy. At autopsy, cerebral atrophy with decreased brain weight, inflammatory cells, infiltrate microglial modules, multinucleated cells, attenuation of white matter, and calcification of vessels in the basal ganglia may be seen in HIV infected children. While available evidence indicates that encephalopathy results from infection of the brain, the specific mechanism is unknown. In addition, although some HIV infected children have severe encephalopathy, the degree and course of intellectual and neurological deterioration is variable. Some children are very impaired while others show more intact levels of cognitive development. The time span from the initial HIV infection in the preinatal period to the onset of progressive encephalopathy is not well understood.

Ultmann, et al (10) described developmental abnormalities in 16 patients (seven with AIDS and six with ARC) ages six months to six years. Delayed developmental milestones were seen in both groups. Several children with AIDS lost milestones as their illness progressed. Developmental testing (Bayley Scale and Stanford-Binet) demonstrated more severe cognitive dysfunction in AIDS patients. However, language skills did not show selective deficits. Involvement of the CNS was documented in all patients with AIDS. However, these investigators noted that erratic caretaking and disturbed home environments could have affected their findings.

Epstein, et al (11) found that all nine children with AIDS out of their cohort of 36 children with HIV infection (ages two months to 11 years at the time of initial diagnosis) had some abnormality in developmental assessment. Delays in motor function and expressive speech were more common than delays in receptive speech. Intellectual deterioration was documented in one child.

Although Belman, et al (12) noted CNS dysfunction in 61 of 68 infants with symptomatic HIV infection, the course and pattern of intellectual deterioration was noted to be quite variable. Psychometric evaluations of 45 children, from infancy to school age (28 with AIDS and 17 with ARC) revealed that 38 had cognitive impairments. However, seven children (two with AIDS and five with ARC) functioned normally, 19 children (12 with AIDS and seven with ARC) functioned within the borderline or mild range of mental retardation, and 19 children (14 with AIDS and five with ARC) functioned within the moderate to severe range of mental retardation.

Taken together, prior studies indicate a significant impact of HIV infection and AIDS on young children's neurological status and cognitive development. However, the degree of developmental impact and intellectual deterioration reported in prior studies have ranged widely. The broad age span (infancy through school age) used in prior studies limits their applicability to assessing the specific impact of HIV infection and AIDS on infants and young children. Cross sectional studies have provided no information concerning neurodevelopmental course, and small sample sizes have precluded studying factors that influence individual differences in developmental prognosis. In addition, prior studies are limited by the presence of significant environmental disruption. For example, one major population of HIV infected children, children of drug abusing mothers, is very difficult to follow prospectively. The level of family disorganization in AIDS populations also has made it difficult to assess or control for environmental influences on cognitive development. Finally, with the exception of one pilot study with a small sample size (13), no study has assessed HIV infected infants' cognitive development using a measure of visual infant recognition memory which might be expected to be the most sensitive to early cognitive deficits (14, 15).

The proposed study will address several important gaps in scientific knowledge of the neurodevelopmental aspects of HIV infection in infants and young children. By using a prospective study design, the neurodevelopmental consequences of HIV infection and AIDS in infants and young children can be tracked with greater precision than has been possible in prior studies. The proposed study will assess covarying influences on cognitive development which has not been done in prior studies. This research will provide important information concerning individual differences in the neurodevelopmental prognosis of HIV infected infants. Finally, the proposed use of visual infant recognition memory tests a method for earlier, more accurate detection of cognitive deficits in HIV infected infants.

C.   Preliminary Studies
The Uganda Project: Several preliminary studies involving Ugandan children form the basis of this proposal. An initial study at the Kasangati Health Center was conducted by Johnson and Olness in 1984 to assess development with a modified Denver Developmental Screening Test. A special questionnaire to assess maternal concern about various behaviors was translated into the Luganda language.

In 1988, a Program Project Grant was funded by the National Institutes of Health to study transmission and course of HIV infection in Ugandan infants. At this point in time, 1,850 pregnant mothers have been enrolled. Twenty-four percent of these mother have had positive HIV ELISA screening tests documented twice and sera is being held from all women tested for Western Blot confirmation. As of August 1, 1989, 410 babies have been born and are being followed every two weeks at New Mulago Hospital of Makerere University in Kampala, Uganda or in their homes by health visitors. Three abstracts related to work done thus far have been submitted, and one has been accepted for presentation at the Pediatrics Infectious Disease conference in October, 1989 (Abstracts appendix 1)

Collaborative arrangements for these studies have been developed and are functioning well (Memorandum of Understanding appendix 3). Professor Christopher Ndugwa, Chairman of Pediatrics at Makerere University, is the Principle Ugandan Investigator (Letter of Agreement appendix 2). Dr. Laura Guay, Senior Instructor on the CWRU faculty, is the Project Field Officer and coordinates implementation in Uganda. She works closely with Dr. Henry Friesen, Overall Coordinator of Pediatrics AIDS projects in Uganda. Together, they supervise a Pediatric HIV Referral Clinic in operation at Mulago Hospital. Collaborative working relationships have been excellent. Two joint reviews of all program projects have been conducted, one in Uganda and one in Cleveland (Report to NIH appendix 4).

Subject recruitment procedures are now in place. The Obstetrics Clinic at New Mulago Hospital is under the supervision of Professor Mmiro, Chairman of Obstetrics, who is studying the effects of pregnancy on the progression of maternal HIV infection. Weekly meetings are held in Uganda involving Professors Ndugwa, Mmiro, Dr. Friesen, Dr. Guay, and other Ugandan Medical Officers involved in implementing these studies. Baseline neurologic exams are now being conducted on each infant at each pediatric visit. The home visitation follow-up that is so critical to effective follow-up of the population is well in place.

The proposed project brings together an interdisciplinary team of investigators with expertise in areas directly relevant to the proposed study: Karen Olness, M.D., Project Investigator, is a pediatrician who has had extensive experience in clinical, teaching, and research work in developing countries. She is the Principal Investigator on the Vertical Transmission Study of HIV Infection in Ugandan Infants and has coordinated the successful implementation of this study. Previously, she has designed, implemented, and completed two field studies: an epidemiologic survey of immunity to poliomyelitis in the Lao population (16), and an anthropometric survey among children in S.E. Asian refugee camps (17). She is experienced in solving problems inherent in field research and in cross-cultural communication. She has written a manual for field use, Practical Pediatrics in Developing Countries, now in its 5th edition (18). Dennis D. Drotar, Ph.D., Project Co-Investigator, is a psychologist with research and clinical experience in developmental assessment and follow-up studies of the psychological development of infants at risk (19). He has been the Principal Investigator on several NIMH studies of the psychological development of failure to thrive infants. He is experienced in the clinical assessment of infants and analysis of data from prospective studies of cognitive development of infants at risk. Dr. Drotar will supervise the conduct of the cognitive and environment assessments and work closely with the consultant, Joseph F. Fagan, Ph.D., to implement the assessment of visual recognition memory. Dr. Fagan has had extensive experience in research concerning infant recognition memory, in follow-up studies of infant risk populations (14, 15) and application of his method to the assessment of intelligence in young infants, including infants at risk owing to various biologic risk conditions. Dr. Fagan has collaborated with Dr. Drotar on the clinical application of the Fagan test to infants with neurological deficits (20). Consultation on the analysis of data pertaining to the interrelationship of neurological and psychological deficits will be provided by The Rainbow Learning Center (Letter of Agreement appendix 5). <u>Howard R. Hall, Ph.D., Psy.D.</u>, Project Co-Investigator, a clinical and pediatric psychologist with extensive experience in behavioral pediatrics. His research with young children, adolescents, and adults has been in psychoneuroimmunology. He has completed a three month seminar course on international health issues including those of Uganda. He will travel to Uganda to provide on-site supervision of psychometric testing and management of psychologic data. <u>Max Wiznitzer, M.D.</u>, Project Co-Investigator, a pediatric neurologist and developmental pediatrician, will be responsible for the sensorimotor neurologic examination of all subjects. He has served as a pediatric neurologist conducting neurologic evaluations in a study of preschool and school-aged children with developmental language disorders, autism, and mental retardation. He will travel to Uganda twice yearly for on-site supervision of examinations and will review all videotapes of these examinations. <u>David Hom, Ph.D.</u>, the statistics and epidemiology consultant for the proposed project has had experience in working with large scale data sets in epidemiological and field studies. He is managing the data collection and analysis for the Uganda project and is familiar with the issues in data management for the proposed study.

The experience of this investigatory team and the preliminary studies already conducted provide a solid base for the proposed study (relevant recent publications of project investigators and consultants, appendix 6). The feasibility of subject recruitment and securing the necessary sample size has been documented in our follow-up study of infants born to HIV positive mothers that is currently underway. Given the high seroprevalence of HIV infections among women of child bearing age in Uganda, a relatively large sample of infants can be recruited. The continuous care and outreach we have in place will facilitate follow-up and reduce attrition. In addition, the fact that infants are from relatively homogeneous, stable families will enhance our ability to determine the specific effects of the HIV virus on development. Pregnant Ugandan women rarely smoke or take drugs. Furthermore, because of strong cultural commitments to family and villages, it should be easier to assess environments and care than with HIV infected infants in the USA.

D. Experimental Design and Methods

<u>Basic Design</u>: The study design is a prospective follow-up study in which the neurodevelopmental status of two groups of infants will be compared: (1) 320 infants who are HIV positive at birth, and (2) 100 infants who begin the study HIV negative and remain HIV negative. It should be noted that the two groups of infants who are identified as HIV positive versus HIV negative at birth include several subgroups: Some infants who are positive at birth will have passive antibodies and will eventually become HIV negative. Moreover, infants in the HIV positive group who remain infected include two groups: (1) infants who develop clinical symptoms of AIDS and (2) those who remain symptomatic. Finally, some children who are HIV negative at birth will later become HIV positive as shown below:

(N =320)	HIV Positive at Birth	Passive Antibody Become HIV Negative (Group 1) (N = 224) (70%)
		Infected Progress to AIDS (Group 2) (N = 80) (25%)
		Asymptomatic (Group 3) (N = 16) (5%)
(N = 100)	HIV Negative	Remain HIV Negative (Group 4) (N =98) (98%)
		Become HIV Positive (Group 5) (N = 2) (2%)

The proposed design will involve several group comparisons: The primary comparison will be between infants who are HIV positive at birth and who remain infected (Groups 2 and 3) versus infants who are HIV negative at birth and who remain HIV negative (Group 4). This comparison will provide information concerning the effects of HIV infection on cognitive and neurological development. The proposed design also allows for an important comparison within group of the neurodevelopment of two groups of HIV infected infants: Infected infants who develop clinical symptoms of AIDS (Group 2) versus infected infants who remain asymptomatic (Group 3). We anticipate that infants who are born HIV negative and convert to HIV positive (Group 5) will not have sufficient numbers for meaningful analysis in the proposed study.

Subjects: The study population will be drawn from two cohorts of mothers seen at Mulago Hospital of Makerere University in Kampala, Uganda: Mothers who are HIV negative and mothers who are HIV positive. Both cohorts will be from the Baganda tribal group and will reside within the greater Kampala area (7-8 mile radius from the center of Kampala).

1. Selection Criteria: Pregnant Ugandan women who attend the antenatal clinic at New Mulago Hospital will be enrolled if they fulfill the following criteria:
    a. First visit to the antenatal clinic of New Mulago Hospital for this pregnancy.
    b. Residence in the greater Kampala area.
    c. Declared intention to deliver at New Mulago Hospital
    d. Agreement to have blood taken for serologic tests for HIV and, if selected, to participate in the pediatric AIDS study.

2. To reduce the likelihood of the confounding effects of developmental or physical handicaps, and illness-related problems due to problems other than HIV infection, the criteria will also include the following:
    a. Full-term status with no evidence of prematurity.
    b. No evidence of gross neurologic or genetic impairment based on initial newborn exam, e.g. an infant with evidence of Down's syndrome or spina bifida would not be enrolled in this study. (The infant's, maturity, and health of the mother   will be recorded as will complications during delivery and newborn period).

3. Specific Recruitment Procedures: Approximately 12,000 women attend New Mulago antenatal clinical annually, and between 8,000 - 9,000 deliver in the hospital. Our preliminary studies indicate that seropositivity is 24%. Approximately 10,000 women will be screened over a period of two years to obtain a subject pool that is more than adequate to recruit the necessary subjects.

No. screened	10,000
24% HIV seropositive	2,400
80% consent to the study	1,903
70% delivery in hospital	1,331
5% (N=67) Abnormal infants	1,264

Mothers attend the antenatal clinic of New Mulago Hospital to listen to a presentation concerning the study. If they wish to join the study, and declare their intention to deliver at New Mulago Hospital, they are asked to give informed consent for blood drawing from themselves and for their infants following birth. It is explained that not all children from all mothers tested will be enrolled in the study. After consent is obtained, they are counselled with respect to possible HIV infection and they receive an identity card with a study number. The same study number is entered on the antenatal card (Form 1.1 appendix 7).

Research assistants come to the hospital daily to look for the study number on charts of newly delivered mothers. HIV negative mothers will be selected according to a previous computer randomized list of all numbers of mothers enrolled and not yet delivered. For each one month period, the project statistician will identify all study numbers that correspond to positive HIV tests and will then take a random sample from study numbers corresponding to negative HIV results. For every four identified "positive" numbers, one "negative" number will be selected. The statistician will then prepare a list of women whose children are eligible for enrollment in the study. This list will be in numerical order for the combined "positive" and "negative" study numbers and will show study number, name, date of birth, address, and expected date of delivery for each of the identified/selected women.

Forms will be completed for each enrolled infant and its mother by a research assistant. These include age of mother, parity, history of last pregnancy, number of children and their health, health status of both parents, type of delivery, birth weight, and description of any neonatal or maternal difficulties (Form 2.1 appendix 8).

Blood samples will be taken from mothers and infants (if cord blood was not obtained) and infants will be immunized against BCG and polio. Mothers and infants will be taken to their homes (most of which are in surrounding villages) by health visitors who will later be doing home visits. This insures that the exact location of the home will be known.

Laboratory Procedures: As in adults, the major features of diagnoses of HIV infection include: (1) Suspicion of infection based on risk and clinical presentation and (2) confirmation (when possible) by serologic tests. Mother's blood and their infants cord or placental blood will be taken for HIV investigation. If cord or placental blood was not taken at delivery, blood will be taken from the infant by vena puncture.

Maternal serum samples will be obtained at the time of the first prenatal visit and tested by enzyme-linked immunosorbent assay (ELISA) (Cambridge, Boston). Repeatedly reactive samples are analyzed by IgG Western blotting (Dupont, Geneva, Switzerland). Cord blood from the newborn is similarly analyzed. It is to be noted that positive ELISA or western blot tests in the newborn may reflect transplacental transfer of HIV-specific IgG. We will assess whether or not these tests become negative over time, and if there should be any associated neurodevelopmental deficits in children exposed to but not infected by HIV (Group 1). In the study underway, these studies are repeated at three, six and 18 months.

We are also separating lymphocytes from newborn blood samples and storing in a freezer at -20°C in Uganda. These are then transferred to laboratories at Case Western Reserve University where techniques for probing viral nucleic acid are applied. One of these is the PCR assay that involves enzymatic amplification of small quantities of DNA of known sequence. This provides the potential of more precise diagnosis of HIV infectivity in infants prior to their loss of placentally transferred antibodies. In addition to the above laboratory studies, blood from each newborn will be studied for presence of sickle cell hemoglobin and malaria smears will be done at three, six and 18 months. Additional laboratory studies will be carried out as required in the presence of acute illness in study subjects. Results of these will be kept as part of study data for later analysis.

Clinical Assessment of AIDS in Infants: Clinical criteria are based on the World Health Organization's clinical case definition of pediatric AIDS in Africa. Major criteria include fever (temperature higher than 37.5 degrees C) for 15 days during a month; persistent diarrhea (more than two stools a day that took the shape of a container) for 15 days a month; and failure to thrive (weight-for-age ratio below the 10th percentile on the scale of the National Center for Health statistics) for two consecutive months. Minor criteria include generalized lymphadenopathy, oral-pharyngeal candidiasis after the age of six months, pneumonia, and a generalized dermatitis. For this study, we will also use the monthly infant AIDS score as defined by Ryder and colleagues (21). This score provides three points for each major criterion and two points for each minor criterion except dermatitis, which receives one because of the frequency of various nonspecific skin conditions. Any child with a seropositive mother and a cumulative score of ten or more points will be considered to have clinically defined AIDS. Any child who dies during the first year of life whose AIDS score was at least seven and whose mother was seropositive will be considered to have AIDS.

Special Diagnostic Problems: Serodiagnosis of HIV infection in infants and children is very difficult (9, 21, 22). Passively acquired antibodies may persist for a long time. A seropositive child less than 15 months of age generally needs to have other unequivocal clinical or laboratory evidence supporting the diagnosis of HIV infection. However, the sensitivity of diagnostic testing has not been well defined. Negative results obtained with the PCR test as currently used could still lead us to miss initially a substantial number of infected infants (9, 21). However, our plan for repeat laboratory testing and clinical assessments provides a way to identify cases that may initially be missed. As more reliable and valid methods to establish the diagnosis of HIV infection by direct identification of HIV viral products in newborn tissue or measurement of infant-specific immunity virus become available, these methods will be utilized.

Follow-up Procedures: Home Visits - The first home visit will take place three weeks after birth. Data collected will include interim history, newborn examination, and information about the home environment (Forms 3.1, 3.2, 3.3, 3.4 and Form 4, appendice 9 and 10). The first post-natal visit is scheduled at six weeks. (See Table 2 [appendix 12] for schedule of follow-up visits.) If mothers fail to return, they will be visited at home and encouraged to visit the clinics. Inducements to attend include Polaroid photos of mothers and infants, as well as free medications if required. Health visitors will study households every other week for six months and monthly thereafter. They will complete data sheets including weights and head circumference. Their recorded information will be coded and transferred to computers for storage by medical officers each evening. Home visits to study families provide support that is necessary to keep them involved in the study, as well as health monitoring and early identification and treatment of nutrition and health-related problems. During a typical home visit, the mother and visitor spend some time in greeting which is elaborate in the Ugandan culture. In addition, the home visitors evaluate the infant's progress, weigh, and measure the infants, and inquire about the mother's health and general well-being. In some cases, the home visitor will provide nutritional education or recommend additional pediatric evaluation. Our experiences thus far have suggested that the home visits are well accepted and mothers appear to enjoy the contact and support provided.

Plan for Outcome Assessment: As shown in Table 1 (Appendix 11), the proposed outcome assessment plan includes two categories of measures: (1) Primary measures that assess cognitive development (Bayley and Fagan Tests, behavior, language, and neurological status), and (2) Secondary measures that assess covarying factors that may influence cognitive development including children's health and nutritional status, maternal health and neurologic status, family socioeconomic status, structure, and caretaking competence.

As shown in Table 2 (Appendix 12), cognitive development, physical growth, neurologic status, and physical status will be assessed at three month intervals for the first 12 months and at 18 and 24 months. Intensive assessment is needed to detect deterioration in cognitive status. The Fagan Test is the one exception to this plan, for experimental work has been conducted with infants only up to 12 months of age. Caretaking competence and maternal health will be assessed at six month intervals. Assessment of physical growth and family structure will take place during home visits conducted by health visitors.

1. Primary Measures: Cognitive Development
   a. Bayley Scale of Mental Development: The Bayley Scale of Mental Development (Appendix 13) assesses a range of skills demonstrated by infants in many cultures such as sensorimotor ability, memory, vocalization, and problem-solving ability (23). This scale was standardized on a sample of 1,260 children in the U.S.A. which included white and non-white, and urban and rural samples (23). Our experiences in pretesting the Bayley Scale with Ugandan infants suggested that the Bayley Scales can be effectively used in this culture. This scale has been used successfully by investigators in rural Kenya (33). In the U.S., standardized sample, split-half reliability quotients range from .81 to .93 with a median value of .88. Standard errors of measurement range from 4.2 to 6.9 at different ages. Test retest reliability one week (percentage agreement) is 76.4. Interobserver agreement in scoring is relatively high (89%) based on data from a sample of eight month old infants (23). Scores on this instrument correlate highly with other tests such as the Stanford-Binet Form L-M (r=.53 to r=.57) in infants of similar ages 24-30 months (23). The validity of the Bayley Scale in predicting the cognitive development of children whose abilities are in the normal range is questionable (24), but is considered better with infant risk populations suggesting that this instrument will be useful in detecting cognitive deficits in the proposed study.

   Special considerations in administration and scoring: Consistent with experiences of other investigators, we anticipate that some changes will be made in test protocol and scoring to adapt the Bayley Scale to infants in the Ugandan culture and testing conditions. For example, pictures used for labeling and word recognition will be taken from local picture books. Objects that are frequently found in the Ugandan culture will be used for object naming task. Certain test items requiring recognition of unfamiliar objects will be excluded.

   b. Fagan Test of Infant Intelligence (Appendix 14): The Fagan Test assesses visual recognition ability which is not measured by the Bayley Scale. Because performance on the Fagan Test is independent of motoric response, this test may be especially useful in assessing the cognitive abilities of HIV infected infants whose motor-coordination and responsiveness may be affected by neurological deficits (20). Finally, research with several infant risk populations has suggested that the Fagan Test may be especially useful in detecting early neurological dysfunction (14, 15, 24, 25).
   Developed from research that has shown that infants encode, retain, categorize and retrieve visual information, the Fagan Test assesses the infants' (ages 3 - 12 months) ability to process visual information. The Fagan Test is composed of a stage on which a standardized set of pictures are presented for viewing by the infant (see appendix). During testing, the infant sits on a parent's lap to view the pictures placed on the stage. After viewing one picture, the infant is faced with a choice between that picture and a new one. The normal infant will spend more time looking at the new picture. A certified tester records the length of time spent looking at each picture on a user-

friendly computerized scoring system. The Fagan Test is totally non-invasive and takes about 15 minutes to administer. Interrater reliability for the FTII is excellent (.97). Predictive validity derived from studies of normal and handicapped samples has averaged around .50 (25).

Scores on the Fagan test differentiate between groups of normal infants versus those at risk for cognitive deficit (25) and predict intellectual functioning in infants at high risk for later mental retardation (21-26). Scores on the Fagan Test have also identified deficits associated with teratogen exposure in offspring of women exposed to polychlorinated biphenyls (PCB) during pregnancy (27), suggesting that this test can detect cognitive deficits in children associated with central nervous system dysfunction. At least one study has suggested that abnormal scores on the Fagan Test are associated with HIV positive infants who also demonstrated an abnormal neurological exam and deficits in developmental test performance.

2. Behavior during testing: Bayley Infant Behavior Record (IBR): Infants who are exposed to the HIV virus might be expected to demonstrate abnormal behavior severe enough to affect their response to cognitive testing. The Bayley Infant Behavior Record will be used to assess the impact of HIV infection on clinically relevant dimensions of behavior. The Infant Behavior Record (IBR) consists of 30 items that characterize an infant's behavior during the administration of the Bayley Scale of Mental Development (23). The IBR has been used in several normative samples such as the Louisville Twin Study with healthy prematures, as well as high risk prematures (28-31). Psychometric properties of this measure are relatively well documented. The IBR includes 16 items which rate general interpersonal, affective, and motivational behavior on nine point scales, nine that assesses the child's interest in specific modes of sensory experience, and five that record clinical impressions of behavior. Each point of the rating scale is anchored by a behavioral description. Scores on the IBR yield several factors such as affective responsiveness, activity level, or task orientation: Based on previous research, two age-constant factors, Test Affect and Task Orientation will be derived from the IBR (29).

3. Language Assessment: A supplementary assessment of children's language will provide a more comprehensive assessment and language functioning than can be obtained by the Bayley Scale alone. Comprehensive assessment of language development is necessary to sample language abilities that might be expected to be sensitive to the effects of neurological changes during the first two years of life. Using the Sequenced Inventory of Communication (32) as a guide for item inclusion and scoring, we will obtain a sample of the child's spontaneous language. In addition, the child will be asked to respond to several language tasks including imitation of speech, repetition of digits, and response to different comprehension tasks. Several measures will be taken from the language sample including two and three word combinations, verb phrases, questions, and mean length utterance. The specific questions used in the comprehension tasks will be developed in collaboration with Ugandan research staff so that they accurately reflect the child's experience. The language sample will be audiotaped and subsequently analyzed for the response measures. Interrater reliability will be obtained for each response measure.

4. Motor Development: The Bayley Motor Scale will assess motor development. All items will be given with the exception that items requiring stairs will be omitted because stairs are not found in the environment of these children. Psychometric data has been reported for the Bayley Motor Scale that is comparable to that of the Mental Scale (31). For example, observer reliability of scoring is high (93.4) and test-retest reliability adequate (75.3) percentage of agreement. Split half reliability scores for the motor scale range

percentage of agreement. Split half reliability scores for the motor scale range from .78 to .90 in the ages of the proposed study (3-30 months)

5. Neurologic Status
    a.   The neonatal neurologic examination (15) will be used to evaluate sensorimotor function with assessment of higher cortical functions being done within the psychological testing. This will allow for a more efficient use of the examiner's time during trips to the child's home. The neurological exam will assess central and peripheral nervous system function. A baseline evaluation using the Neonatal Neurologic Examination will be done after birth and prior to hospital discharge. This exam emphasizes habituation, movement and tone, reflexes and neurobehavioral reactivity. Each item will be graded in four to five steps and is marked on the scoring sheet. Since items are state dependent, the neonate's state will be recorded with each test item (Dubowitz exam page appendix 15).

    b.   Sensorimotor function during the first year of life will be tested using the neurologic evaluation developed by Amiel-Tison (35). Items testing sensation, standing and walking will be added. This evaluation will be sensitive to changes in tone and primitive reflexes that reflect sensorimotor dysfunction in children with HIV infections. This scale can also identify peripheral nerve and muscle dysfunction because of the hypotonia and decreased motor function in the latter. Each item is easily scored using the form developed by Amiel-Tison. Testing will be rescheduled if the infant is acutely ill and uncomfortable or agitated. Because a wide range of individual variations in tone are present in normal development, a persistent pattern of abnormality over serial examinations and present at one year must be present before the findings will be classified as abnormal. This pattern will allow us to identify the time of appearance of early changes in the sensorimotor examination as well as the identification of transient neuromotor abnormalities (Amiel-Tison Exam appendix 16).

    The sensorimotor examination for the second year of life will encompass the following functional groups: Gross motor skills; Fine motor skills; Tone and posture; Involuntary movements; Sensory; and Cranial nerves. Right and left sided function will be separately scored. Each test will be scored as 0 = normal, 1 = mild-moderately abnormal, and 2 = severely abnormal (Toddler Neurologic Exam appendix 17).

    The sensorimotor neurologic examination will be performed by the local medical officer in the project, who will be trained in the administration of the examination by a pediatric neurologist. Training will be done on the neurologist's initial visit to Uganda and will be verified on subsequent trips and by the neurologist's evaluation of videotaped examinations. Instructions on examination administration is available in publications by Dubowitz and Amiel-Tison, on a videotape of the infant and toddler exam and in a manual for the older child's exam. Independent scoring of the videotape and supervised exams will be done to enhance inter-observer reliability.

    Cross-cultural application of measures: The measures were chosen for their relative ease of administration, feasibility for use in the field, and potential transfer across cultures. The Fagan test is portable, can be adapted for field use by using a hand held recorder and has been utilized in home settings in several studies. The Fagan test assesses visual recognition memory, a function which can readily be assessed across different cultures. This test has been used in Sweden and Egypt, as well as with black and white infants in the USA. Alternate forms of the test for black infants will be used in this study.

The Bayley Scale of Mental Development has been utilized in several different cultures outside the USA, including with Kenyan infants (33). Some of the Bayley items involve demonstration of actions such as putting cubes in a cup, imitation of actions, or spontaneous exploration such as ringing a bell that will require little change from the standard administration. On the other hand, items involving comprehension of instructions or language related items will require administration of the items in the Ugandan language. The assessors will be trained to administer the items using translations of English to Luganda. To enhance reliability of scoring, infants language will be audiotaped. Picture vocabulary items and objects that are frequently encountered in the Ugandan culture will be substituted for these items based on consultation with health visitors and project staff. While no norms exist for Ugandan infants on the Bayley Test, our plan to compare overall scores of HIV positive versus HIV negative infants from the same culture, should provide a valid comparison. In addition, several prior studies in Ugandan and African infants have indicated that developmental assessments are applicable to this population (33, 36, 37).

Procedures to enhance reliability and consistency of measures in the field: Research staff will be trained in the assessment procedures which will include: (1) Introduction and background including readings, (2) Observation of the procedures and supervised practice and administration with the Project Co-investigators and Consultants. Once in the field, procedures will be videotaped and sent back for review. Project investigators will assess the reliability of test administration, the degree of change or drift in procedures over time, and use this information to correct errors in test administration. Videotapes of the cognitive and neurologic assessments will be done on five children at 3, 6, 9, 12, 18 and 24 months. Reliability of administration and scoring of the developmental tests and neurological exam will be assessed by comparing test administration of the research staff from videotapes with the Project Investigators' scoring of the same tasks. Problems in administration will be managed by project investigators who will visit the research site to meet with the research staff to trouble-shoot procedures and correct errors in administration.

Neurological exams will be conducted by a physician who will be trained by the project Co-investigator. Assessments of cognitive development (Bayley Infant Behavior Record, Fagan Test, Language Assessment) and home observations will be conducted by trained research assistants who are familiar with Ugandan language and culture. All staff who conduct assessments will not have information about mother or child's HIV status, but we recognize that maternal health status will be obvious to home visitors. The physicians who conduct the neurological assessment will not have information about the child's cognitive assessment. Research assistants who conduct the cognitive assessments will not have information about the neurological assessments. Cognitive and neurological assessments will be conducted in separate home visits.

6. Secondary Measures: Assessment of Covarying Influences
   a.   Children's Nutritional Status: We plan to limit the confounding effects of malnutrition due to illnesses other than AIDS and assess the effects of malnutrition in several ways: First, in contrast to other Ugandan infants, infants in the proposed study will receive intensive health monitoring by the home visitor, preventive health care including

immunizations, and ready access to pediatric diagnosis and treatment by the study pediatrician. The close monitoring of children's physical growth and health will identify changes in growth patterns and health as soon as they become evident and allow our medical staff to institute nutritional and medical treatment before these problems become serious or chronic. Medical treatment is readily available for children who suffer from acute malnutrition, and food is available through the resources of the Save the Children Fund. We anticipate that the severe and prolonged malnutrition that pose the most serious hazard to cognitive development would be prevented by health monitoring and access to treatment would, thus, not pose a significant threat to study validity. In addition, our intensive monitoring of nutrition and children's health at close intervals will allow us to assess the impact of changes in children's nutritional status and physical health, including the onset and duration of periods of malnutrition that does occur, including malnutrition that is a concomitant of HIV infection.

b.   Assessment Procedures: Standard anthropometric measures of weight and length will be used to assess malnutrition. Forms from the US National Center for Health Statistics that are reflected in the Road to Health Chart that is used routinely in Uganda Maternal-Child Health Clinics will be used to assess weight for height ratios. In addition, clinical signs of malnutrition such as lightening of hair roots, increased ear elasticity, bitot's spots in the eyes, cracked mouth corners, "enameled" skin as commonly present in kwashiorkor, and edema, will be recorded.

Severe malnutrition will be defined as weight and height below the fifth percentile in association with two or more clinical signs and requirement for hospitalization. Moderate malnutrition includes weight and height below the fifth percentile in association with one or more clinical signs and responds to ambulatory treatment. Mild malnutrition will be defined as those children below the fifth percentile for weight and height with no clinical signs of malnutrition. Weight for height (resting) and height for age (38) will also be used to assess nutritional status.

c.   Children's Health Status: Child health will be assessed by physical examination during well-child visits and by the home visitor's assessments. Children's symptoms, illnesses, and treatments will be documented (See Form, appendix 9).

d.   Maternal Health and Neurological Status: We anticipate that some mothers will develop illness and/or cognitive impairment significant enough to affect the level of caretaking provided to the child. By assessing maternal health and neurological status over time, we will determine individual differences in course and severity of maternal illness, identify cases in which the maternal health is severely affected and the point at when this occurred. Second, our prospective assessment of the number and type of caretakers and caretaking competence will document the variance in cognitive outcomes accounted for by deterioration in the quality of.the child's caretaking owing to maternal illness or death.

1.   Assessment of Maternal Health: General and systemic examination will assess presence of major and minor signs of AIDS as defined by the WHO. Besides HIV tests, these mothers will be tested for malaria parasites, syphilis and anemia. Routine urinalysis and hemoglobin test will be done at study entry. Mothers will be monitored for anemia, rashes, BP, oral thrush, and

PV discharge during their pregnancy. Subsequent visits will be carried out monthly in early pregnancy, fortnightly between the 28th and 36th weeks and weekly thereafter. Mothers and children will be seen initially at postnatal clinic. Maternal health and neurological status will be assessed at six month intervals.

2. The children's mothers will be screened for dementia and motor deficits secondary to HIV infection using the Micro Neurological History and Examination developed by Richard Price, M.D. (University of Minnesota), and used by the AIDS Clinical Trials Group in their studies. This screen, which requires 10-15 minutes, tests for memory, concentration, and motor dysfunction (6) and will be given yearly. Women with abnormal results will be referred for more detailed evaluation by a local neurologist (ACTG Micro Neurologic Exam appendix 18).

7. Family Socioeconomic Status and Home Environment: Using a classification schema based on prior research concerning the impact of nutrition and environment on child development (39-42), several different types of environmental factors will be assessed:

a. Socioeconomic status: Measures will include: Family income (gross family and per capita), parental education, number of years of schooling, and parental literacy.

b. Family environment and structure: Parental marital status, family structure, changes in family structure, household density (ratio of number of rooms in the house to number of people living in the house), general sanitary conditions of the home, and possessions of parent and child will be assessed at three months intervals using home visits. Measures of general sanitary conditions in the home including the nature of the water supply, cooking utensils, etc., are currently being gathered as a part of the Uganda project (See appendix 10)

c. Number and types of caretakers: The number and type of caretakers (mother, extended family, and siblings) that are involved in the child's care, and the approximate distribution of time that the child is taken care of by different family members will be assessed by home observation procedures.

d. Caretaking competence: Based on procedures developed by Sigman, et al (33) to observe maternal-child interactions in Kenya, the following behaviors will be observed using a time sampling procedure for a 30 minute period for the mother or major caretaker.
Physical care: Caregiving behavior such as feeding, washing, changing clothes.
Hold/carry: Holding in arms or on lap, picking-up or carrying so that the child's feet are off the ground.
Touch: Touching any part of the child.
Social interaction: Caregiver and child is actively involved in an ongoing social interchange.
Talks to toddler: Talking directly to the child while looking at the child or holding the child and interacting.
Responses to vocalization/distress: Vocal physical response to child vocalization or cries within five seconds.
Inter-observer reliability data will be gathered on the observational data using videotaped observations. A prior field study using a similar observational procedure yielded high inter-rater reliability (majority of measures above .90) (33). Preliminary validity has been obtained for similar interactional measures in Kenyan toddlers (33).

8.　Data Analysis: The first phase of data analysis will include data reduction. The second phase will include four analytic steps: (1) descriptive analyses, (2) analyses of major hypotheses involving the comparison of the neurodevelopment of HIV positive versus HIV negative infants, (3) analyses of factors that predict the deterioration in neurodevelopment, (4) analyses of the effect of covariates on cognitive development.

　　a.　Data reduction of primary measures: The total number of items passed will be used in subsequent analyses of data from the Bayley Scales (Mental and Motor). Scores will not be converted into developmental quotients because the standardization data for the Bayley Scale is not appropriate for this sample. The total number of items passed will be used rather than the highest item passed (ceiling level) because the ordering of items may not be the same for Ugandan as it is for Western toddlers. The Fagan test yields a score which reflects the mean percentage of response to a novel stimulus achieved by infants at a certain age (see description of Fagan test). For example, if an infant were shown a new and previously seen pattern and devoted 10 seconds of looking time to the new pattern and six seconds to the old pattern, this percentage would be 10/16 or 63% for that problem. The sum of these percentages to novelty divided by the number of problems yield a mean novelty preference score for each infant (26). Data from several studies indicate a mean novelty percentage score of lower than 53% is predictive of subsequent cognitive deficiency (mental retardation) (24-27). A mean percentage response to novelty score of 53% or less will be classified as abnormal; scores above this level will be classified as normal. For the Bayley Scale, a score of more than two standard deviations equivalent to a Mental Development Index (MDI) of 68 on U.S. norms will be classified as abnormal.

　　　　Data from the IBR scales will be factor analyzed. Factor scores for two variables: Test Affect and Task Orientation will be used in subsequent analyses. In addition, abnormal test behavior will be scored and tabulated. Abnormal test behaviors are defined as those that have been identified in prior research as infrequently observed in normal infants (24). Detailed item analyses have indicated sharp discontinuity in the distribution of IBR items that are relatively unchangeable across ages (29).

　　　　Data from the language assessment will be reduced as follows: The number of correct responses on the language comprehension tasks will be summed. In addition, a composite measure of language expression will be developed at each age based on several measures, including the number of verbalizations and mean length utterance (33).

　　b.　Data reduction of secondary measures: Nutritional status data will be summarized in several ways. Children's weight and length will be plotted on growth charts. Individual children who demonstrate weight, length, or weight and length below the 5th percentile will be identified. Based on Waterlow (38), two additional indices of nutritional status will be derived: The percentage of weight for height from which a measure of wasting will be derived (reflective of acute nutritional deficits) and a measure of length for age from which a measure of stunting or chronic malnutrition will be derived. Finally, an overall score of malnutrition-related symptoms will be developed based on clinical symptoms.

　　　　Maternal neurological status will be rated as normal versus abnormal. Several measures of family environmental status will be derived including: Stability of caretaking; the number of changes in caretakers; frequency of caretaker's interactions with infants in each observational category; and the overall frequency of caretakers interactions with the child.

c.   Descriptive Analyses: Means, standard deviations, and the distribution for each outcome measure will be tabulated. The frequency of infants who demonstrate abnormal cognitive test performance (on the Bayley and Fagan Tests), abnormal neurological exam, and/or abnormal behavior on the IBR will be tabulated for the entire sample and the HIV positive and HIV negative groups at each age group. Additional scores will be generated by summarizing the pattern of the child's performance over time. For example, children with consecutive normal and abnormal neurological exams will be identified.

d.   Analyses of the neurodevelopmental status of HIV positive and HIV negative infants: Multivariate analyses of variance will be used to assess the significance of differences in cognitive test performance between HIV positive and HIV negative infants on measures of cognitive status (language, developmental, and behavior). We anticipate that these analyses will reveal a significant Group x Time interaction reflecting the deterioration in cognitive test performance of the HIV positive infants across time.

Chi-Square Tests will compare the frequency of infants in each group at each age who have an abnormal test performance on the Fagan Test (mean of 53% or less response to novelty), Bayley Scale and neurological test exam. Log-linear regression analyses will be used to test the differences in the frequency of children in the HIV positive versus HIV negative group who demonstrate abnormal test performance at different ages.

e.   Analyses of developmental test performance in HIV infected children: Additional analyses will assess individual differences in cognitive status over time and the concurrent and predictive relationship of cognitive and neurological status to disease progression. Children who demonstrate progression from HIV positive state to AIDS will be identified. Chi-square and Log-linear regression analyses will be used to determine the relative efficacy of the Fagan versus Bayley Test at three months of age in predicting: (1) subsequent progression to AIDS and (2) change from normal to abnormal neurological exam.

To determine the relationship of initial test performance to subsequent outcomes, performance on the Fagan test and the Bayley Scale at 3, 6, and 9 months will be correlated with scores on the Bayley Scale and Language assessments at 12, 18, and 24 months. Hierarchical regression analyses (43) will determine the relative strength of the Bayley Scale and Fagan test at three to nine months in predicting subsequent Bayley and Language assessment scores at 12, 18, and 24 months. Finally, the relative efficiency of the Bayley versus the Fagan test (sensitivity and specificity) at 3 to 9 months in predicting normal versus abnormal test performance and abnormal neurological exams at 12, 18, and 24 months of age in HIV infected infants will be assessed.

f.   Analysis of confounding or intervening factors: Several different analyses will be used to assess the impact of the following factors on cognitive development: Child nutritional status, maternal health and neurological status, socioeconomic status, stability of caretakers, and caretaking competence. Following data reduction we will determine whether the two major study groups, HIV negative versus HIV positive, differ on any of the covariates using analysis of variance for continuous data and chi square for categorical data. In the event that group differences are identified, analyses of covariance will be used to test the major hypothesis of group differences between HIV positive versus HIV negative infants controlling for the effects of significant covariates.

Correlations will also be computed between various sets of potential covariate variables (e.g., child's nutritional status, maternal neurologic status, caretaking competence, family demographics) and each of the primary outcome measures. Next, hierarchial regression analysis will be conducted to assess the variance in Bayley, language, and IBR scores accounted for by these variables. Finally, hierarchial regression analyses will assess the effects of disease status (HIV positive versus HIV negative) on cognitive outcomes adjusting for the influence of significant covariates.

g.   Sample Attrition: We anticipate two sources of attrition: (1) attrition due to unavailability of subjects for follow-up, and (2) attrition due to death. Our experience suggests that our follow-up program will minimize attrition due to subject unavailability. All infants receive comprehensive pediatric follow-up every two weeks at new Mulago Hospital of Makerere University of Kampala, Uganda or in their homes by health visitors. Thus far in the Uganda project, outreach follow-up has resulted in minimal (less than 5%) attrition due to subject unavailability. We anticipate that we will be able to maintain a low level of attrition (5%) for the proposed project.

Based on WHO statistics, we anticipate a mortality rate of 5% for the Uganda population due to non-AIDS-related causes. This may be a conservative estimate because this sample will receive excellent health care relative to community standards. We anticipate significant levels of mortality due to AIDS. A study of perinatal transmission of the HIV virus to infants of seropositive women in Zaire indicated a 6.2% compared to 1.2% death rate in the first 28 days of life for HIV positive infants and 21% mortality (compared to 3.8% controls) overall for the first year of life (21). We anticipate similar rates of attrition in the proposed study. Taken together, our projected rates of attrition to sample unavailability (5%) and infant mortality (20%) yield a total attrition rate of 25% for one year for HIV positive infants. We estimate an attrition rate of 40% in HIV positive infants by age two. We anticipate an attrition rate of 10% (5% from subject unavailability and 5% mortality) per year in the HIV negative group. If more reliable laboratory methods for diagnosis of early HIV infection in infants become available, we will be able to enroll fewer HIV positive infants.

9.   Sample Size/Power Considerations: The proposed sample size was selected to ensure that there would be adequate power to detect differences among the groups, allowing for attrition due to mortality and incomplete follow-up. We have based sample size requirements on medium size effects because we believe that the regressive changes previously established in AIDS patients will be quite easy to document.

Our sample size includes 100 infants who are HIV negative and 320 infants who are HIV positive. Based on projected attrition, this would yield a sample size of 90 HIV negative and 240 HIV positive infants for the first year analysis. Of the 240 HIV positive infants, approximately 60% will seroconvert to HIV negative status, leaving approximately 96 HIV positive infants for comparative analysis. Power calculations for the first year analyses are as follows: Based on Cohen (44), we anticipate a power of .90 to detect medium effect size (f = .25) at p < .05 using analysis of variance. To detect a medium effect size using chi-square analysis at p < .05, the power is .90. Analyses of power for the multiple regression analysis assumes that the number of independent variables will be five or less and is calculated to detect a moderate effect size

r^2 ~.16. The power is above .90 for the entire sample and .80 for the HIV positive group.

At two year follow-up, we anticipate a total of 40% attrition in the HIV positive group and 20% in the HIV negative group. This would yield a total number of 80 HIV negative infants and 57 HIV positive infants for the two year analyses. Power for analysis of variance to test group differences would be .83 to detect a small to medium effect size ($f = .20$) at $p < .05$. The power for chi-square analyses to detect a medium to large effect size ($f = .40$) is .80. Finally, the power for regression analyses at age two (assuming the number of independent variables are five or less) and calculated to detect a medium effect size $r^2 = .20$) is above .95 for the entire sample and .80 for the HIV positive group.

10.   Collaborative Arrangements and Data Management: The study will be conducted by the Departments of Pediatrics and Child Health and Obstetrics and Gynecology of Makerere University, in collaboration with Case Western Reserve University and under the national coordination of AIDS activities in Uganda by the AIDS Control Program. The process of enrollment and follow-up will be identical for the Core Study already underway and for the proposed neurodevelopmental follow-up study. Wherever possible, resources and staff will be shared. Laboratory facilities already in-place in Uganda and Cleveland will provide data not only to the core study but to three other studies that are part of the Program Project. The proposed study will require its own field coordinator with special expertise in carrying out proposed psychometric and neurologic exams as well as recording of that data. Because some of these exams will be better carried out at home, it will necessitate additional home visits and, therefore, will require purchase or rental of its own vehicle and a driver for that purpose.

Arrangements have been made with the Entebbe Data Center to accommodate necessary data collection, entry and storage in their system. Contact will be through on-site visits to Entebbe (Dr. Hom will visit Uganda in year 1 of the Program) and mail (including electronic mail) and telephone communications.

The core unit will maintain a core data base of survey data from Entebbe that will be available to each project. Data will be transferred in computer readable format. Copies of a sample of paper records will also be sent for quality control evaluations of data entry. The proposed project will have a data base on the VAX. A programmer attached to the core will provide programming support for each project and the core data base.

11.   Data Management: Data from the ongoing pediatric study are currently being maintained and managed on a Zenith 286 processor laptop computer with storage capacity of 20 megabytes. A Ugandan data analyst and programmer with a MS in statistics from the University of Guelph, Canada, currently performs data entry and management of all projects in Uganda with supervision and program development provided by the Data Management Center in the Case Western Reserve University, Department of Epidemiology and Biostatistics.

All current data has been entered on the CDC developed program Epi-Info (Version 3.0), with additional database management and file manipulation provided by dBase IV (Ashton-Tate). Simplicity of the program Epi-Info in combination with the sophisticated dBase IV program allows data entry and management to be accomplished quickly and accurately. Individual screen data-entry for each form, minimizing opportunity for data entry error, is being used in Epi-Info. Study participant linkage between studies and between forms (Antenatal and delivery data forms) are being accomplished with dBase IV.

All entry programs and quality control measures were generated by the Data Management Center with suggested revisions provided by the resident programmer. Data files archival and back-up is performed routinely on a weekly basis. Transfer of data to computers maintained at CWRU is accomplished on a routine basis by courier to insure quality control and to allow for additional statistical analysis. All analyses are being accomplished using SPSS-PC+ (Version 3), in addition to complex analyses being performed on the Biometry Computer (VAX 11/750 computer). A larger tabletop computer (AT&T 636 WGS) (20 MH$_z$ 386 processor with 80 megabytes of disk space) has been acquired and is currently being installed with all pertinent programs for analysis and data management in Uganda. Shipment of this computer to Uganda is currently being arranged.

12. Time Line of Project Activities: The projected time line for implementation of study activities is shown below:

TIME LINE OF PROJECT ACTIVITIES

1-3 months	3 months	6 months	12 months	24 months	30 months	36 months
Training of research assistants. Begin refinement of measures. Subject recruitment already in place. Obtain consent.	Begin collection of cognitive & neurological data.	Complete refinement of measures.	Subject enrollment complete.	All infants complete one year follow-up assessment	Complete research reports on one year outcome data.	All infants complete two year follow-up assessment. Begin analysis of two year outcome data.

Training of research assistants in the administration of measures and consent for family participating will be obtained during the first three months of the study. Procedures for subject recruitment are already well in place. Data collection will begin at three months and continue to age 30 months. We anticipate that our sample will be enrolled in the study within 12 months. Additional refinement of the Bayley Scale and language assessment will be completed by six months, and before these measures are needed. Initial data reduction and analysis based on the first year outcome data will begin at 24 months and will be after the start of the project and completed by 30 months. Data collection will be completed by 36 months.

13. Human Subjects: This project will assess neurodevelopmental progress in a cohort of Ugandan children who are already being followed with respect to their HIV status.

a. Population description: These studies will compare several groups of infants born to mothers at the New Mulago Hospital in Kampala, Uganda and who reside within the greater Kampala area. These studies include infants who are HIV positive at birth and progress to clinical AIDS, infants who are HIV positive at birth but test negative after one year, and a infants who are negative at birth and remain negative. Information obtained from the blood studies is already being obtained for a previously approved study of vertical transmission of AIDS from Ugandan mothers to their infants.

The proposed study will evaluate neurologic and neuro-developmental parameters in these infants starting at three months and continuing at three month intervals through 18 months and six month intervals thereafter. Infants will be visited in their homes every two weeks for the first six months of the study and monthly thereafter. Follow-up clinic visits occur at six weeks, three, six nine, 12, 18, and 24 months.

1.   <u>Historical information</u> - Data regarding birth history, intercurrent illness, treatments, results of physical examinations, and immunizations will be collected and maintained on medical records. Data regarding family structure and number and patterns of caretaking will be obtained during home visits.

2.   <u>Blood sampling</u> - The initial blood samples will be obtained from cord blood. Subsequent blood testing will be repeated at three, six, and 18 months and will require 7 ml of blood drawn by venipuncture by a physician during the clinic visits. This study will require no blood testing beyond that already defined for the overall vertical transmission study.

3.   <u>Neurodevelopmental testing</u> - This will include routine neurologic assessment, Bayley Scales of Infant Development, Fagan Test of Infant Intelligence, language assessment and behavior ratings.

b.   <u>Recruitment and Consent</u>: Mothers who attend the antenatal clinic of New Mulago Hospital will be invited in groups by Ugandan Health Visitors into an adjoining conference room to hear a presentation regarding the study. If they are willing to join the study and declare their intention to deliver at New Mulago Hospital, they will be asked to give informed consent for blood drawing from themselves and for their infants following birth. It will be explained that not all children from all mothers tested will be enrolled in the study. It is also explained that those enrolled in the study will receive a ride home from the obstetrics unit following discharge. After consent is obtained, they will be counselled with respect to possible HIV infection, and they receive an identity card with a study number. The same study number will be entered on the antenatal card.

c.   <u>Potential Risks</u>: The neurodevelopmental assessments have no known risks. Venipuncture has the minimal risk of slight pain and/or bruising at the site. The volume of blood is small in relation to the total blood volume in this age group and has been demonstrated in numerous prior studies to cause no harm to the subjects.

d.   <u>Precautions to minimize potential risks</u>: Blood will be drawn by an experienced pediatrician, thus minimizing the slight pain of the procedure and risk of local bruising. Data will be available only to study personnel, identified by ID number, thus maintaining confidentiality. Families may choose to withdraw from the study at any time without compromising their further care at Mulago Hospital.

e.   <u>Risk - Benefit Ratio</u>: The importance of determining the neurodevelopmental consequences of HIV infection have been described in the body of the grant. The potential benefits, therefore, seem to outweigh the minimal risk associated with venipuncture. The close monitoring of infants in this study may actually prevent illnesses (e.g. malnutrition) or facilitate earlier treatment.

REFERENCES

1. Mann, J.M.: The global AIDS situation. World Health Stat Quar, 40:185-192, 1987.

2. Widy-Wirski, R., Berkley, S., Downing, R., et al.: Evaluation of the WHO clinical case definition for AIDS in Uganda. JAMA, 260:3286-3289, 1988.

3. Blanche, S., Rouzioux, C., Moscato, M.G., et al.: A prospective study of infants born to women seropositive for human immunodeficiency virus type 1. N Eng J Med, 320:1643-1648, 1989.

4. Minkoff, H, Nandu, D, Menez, R, Fikrig, S.: Pregnancies resulting in infants with acquired immuno-deficiency syndrome or AIDS-related complex: Follow-up of mothers, children, and subsequently born siblings. Obstet Gynecol, 69:288-291, 1987.

5. Novick, LF, Berns, D, Stricof, R, et al.: HIV seroprevalence in newborns in New York State. JAMA, 265:1745-1750, 1989.

6. Price, R.W., Brew, B., Sidtis, J., et al.: The brain in AIDS: Central nervous system HIV-1 infection and AIDS dementia complex. Science, 239:586-592, 1988.

7. Navia, B.A. Price, R.W.: The acquired immunodeficiency syndrome dementia complex as the presenting or sole manifestation of human immunodeficiency virus infection. Arch Neurol, 44:65-69, 1987.

8. Grant, I., Atkinson, J.H., Hesselink, J.R., et al.: Evidence for early central nervous system involvement in the acquired immunodeficiency syndrome (AIDS) and other human immunodeficiency virus (HIV) infections. Ann Internal Med, 107:828-836, 1987.

9. Falloon, J., Eddy, J., Wiener, L., et al.: Human immunodeficiency virus infection in children. J Pediatr, 114:1-30, 1989.

10. Ultmann, M.H., Belman, A.L., Ruff, H.A., et al.: Developmental abnormalities in infants and children with acquired immune deficiency syndrome (AIDS) and AIDS related complex. Develop Med Child Neurol., 27:563-571, 1985.

11. Epstein, L.G., Charer, L.R., Oleske, J.M., et al.: Neurologic manifestations of human immunodeficiency virus in children. Pediatrics, 78:678-687, 1986.

12. Belman, A.L., Diamond, G., Dickson, D., et al.: Pediatric acquired immunodeficiency syndrome: neurologic syndromes. Am J Dis Child, 142:29-35, 1988.

13. Swales, T.P.: Neurocognitive functioning among infants exposed perinatally to HIV infection. Presented at 5th international conference on AIDS, Montreal, 1989.

14. Fagan, J.F., Montie, J.E.: Identifying infants at risk for mental retardation: A cross validation study. Jour Develop Behav Peds, 7:199-200, 1986.

15. Fagan, J.F., McGrath, S.K.: Infant recognition memory and later intelligence. Intelligence, 51:121-130, 1981.

16. Olness, K., Halstead S., Snitbahn, R.: Poliomyelitis in Laos, immunity and epidemiological survey. J Pediatr, August, 1966.

17. Olness K., Yip, R., Indritz, A., Torjesen, E.: An anthropometric study of 1650 Southeast Asian children: Adaptation of growth standards. Am J Dis Child, 138:544-47, 1984.

18. Olness K.: Practical pediatrics in less developed countries: A manual for physicians and physician's assistants. Fifth ed., Minnesota International Health Volunteers, Minneapolis, 1988. Fourth ed., The Garden, Eden Prairie, MN, 1980. Third ed., University of Minnesota Medical School, Minneapolis, 1976.

19. Drotar, D. Sturm, L.A.: Prediction of intellectual development in young children with early histories of nonorganic failure to thrive. J Pediatr Psychol, 13:281-296, 1988.

20. Drotar, D., Mortimer, J., Shepherd, A., Fagan, J.F.: Case report: Recognition memory as a method to assess intelligence in an infant with quadriplegia. Develop Med Child Neurology, 31:391-394, 1989.

21. Ryder, R.W., Wato, N., Hassig, et al.: Perinatal transmission of the human immunodeficiency virus type 1 to infants of seropositive women in Zaire. N Engl J Med, 320:1637-1642, 1989.

22. Katz, S.L., Wilbert, C.M.: Human immunodeficiency virus infection of newborns. N Engl J Med, 320:1687-1688, 1989.

23. Bayley, N: Bayley Scales of Mental Development, New York: Psych. Corp., 1969.

24. Fagan, J.F., Singer, L. T., Montie, J., Shepherd, P.A.: Selective screening device for the early detection of normal or delayed cognitive development in infants at risk for later mental retardation. Pediatrics, 78:1021-1026, 1986.

25. Fagan, J.F., Singer, L.T.: Infant recognition memory as a measure of intelligence. In L.P. Lipsitt (Ed.), Advances in Infancy Research, 2:31-78, 1983.

26. Fagan, J.F., Shepherd, P.A.: The Fagan Test of Infant Intelligence: Training Manual. Infatest Corp.: Cleveland, Ohio, 1986.

27. Jacobson, S.W., Fein, O., Jacobson, J., Schwartz, P., Donler, J.: The effect of intrauterine PCB exposure on visual recognition memory. Child Develop, 56:853-60, 1985.

28. Meisels, S. J., Cross, D, Plunkett, S.W.: Use of the Bayley Infant Behavior record with preterm and fullterm infants, Develop Psychol, 23:473-482, 1987.

29. Wolf, A.W., Lozoff, B.: A clinically interpretable method for analyzing the Bayley Infant Behavior Record. J Pediatr Psychol, 10:199-214, 1985.

30. Matheny, A.P. Jr.: Bayley's Infant Behavior Record: Behavioral components and twin analyses. 51:1157-1167, 1983.

31. Matheny, A.P., Dolan, A.B., Wilson, R.S.: Bayley's Infant Behavior Record: Relations between behaviors and mental test scores. Develop Psychol, 10:606-701, 1981.

32. Hedrick, D.L., Prother, E.M., Tobin, A.R.: Sequenced inventory of communication development expressive and receptive scales. University of Washington Press: Seattle, Washington, 1975.

33. Sigman, M., Neumann, L., Carter, E., Cattle, D.J., D. Souza, S., Biwilbo, N.: Home interactions and the development of Embu toddlers in Kenya. Child Develop, 59:1251-1261, 1989.

34. Dubowitz, L., Dubowitz, V.: The neurological assessment of the preterm and fullterm newborn infant. Clinics Develop Med, No. 79, William Heinemann Medical Books, 1981.

35. Amiel-Tison, C., Grenier, A.: <u>Neurological assessment during the first year of life</u>. Oxford University Press: Oxford, New York, 1986.

36. Geber, M., Dean R.F.A.: Gesell tests on African children. Pediatrics, 20:1055-1065, 1957.

37. Evans, J.L.: <u>Children in Africa: A review of psychological research</u>. Teachers College Press: Columbia University, New York, NY, 1970.

38. Waterlow, J.C.: Classification and definition of protein-calorie malnutrition. Brit Med J, 3:566-569, 1972.

39. Politt, E., Leibel, R.: Biological and social correlates of failure to thrive. In L. Green, E. Johnston, <u>Social & Biological Predictors of Nutritional Status, Physical, Neurological Development</u>. Academic Press: New York, New York, 1986.

40. Christian, N., Mora M.G., Herrera, P.: Family-social characteristics related to the growth of children. Brit J Prev Soc Med, 29:121-130, 1975.

41. Christiansen, N., Voori, Mora, Wagner, M.: Social environment as it relates to malnutrition and mental development. In J. Craviot, L. Hambraeus, B. Vahlquist, <u>Early Nutrition and Mental Development</u>. Swedish Nutritional Foundation: Uppsala, 1974.

42. Richardson, S.A.: <u>Ecology of malnutrition, non-nutritional factors influencing intellectual and behavioral development in nutrition, the nervous system and behavior</u>. WHO Pub 25: Washington, D.C., 1972.

43. Cohen, J., Cohen, P.: <u>Applied Multiple Regression and Correlation Analyses for the Behavioral Sciences</u>. Erlbaum: Hillsdale, New Jersey, 1975.

44. Cohen, J.: <u>Statistical Power Analyses for the Behavioral Sciences</u>. Academic Press: New York, New York, 1977.

Appendix B
Budget Justification

DD   Principal Investigator/Program Director *(Last, first, middle):* _____

DETAILED BUDGET FOR INITIAL BUDGET PERIOD DIRECT COSTS ONLY	FROM 4/1/89	THROUGH 3/31/90

PERSONNEL *(Applicant organization only)*		TYPE APPT. *(months)*	% EFFORT ON PROJ.	INST. BASE SALARY	DOLLAR AMOUNT REQUESTED *(omit cents)*		
NAME	ROLE ON PROJECT				SALARY REQUESTED	FRINGE BENEFITS	TOTALS
	Principal Investigator	12	60*				
	(CU + PI)						
For detailed budget please see page 5.							
*20% contributed, 40% see consortium							
The salary from the	University consortium represents 40% of Dr.						
combined salary from	University and						
SUBTOTALS ⟶					230,094	55,221	285,315

CONSULTANT COSTS

Psychologist	600	Vision Specialist	400	
Audition Specialist	300	Travel for Consultants	1000	2,300

EQUIPMENT *(Itemize)*

Teller Acuity Cards	1050	
Tympanometer	2500	
PC Hardware	2000	5,550

SUPPLIES *(Itemize by category)*

New Jersey Office	2800	
Audiometry Eq. Replacement Parts	500	
Tympanometer Supplies	150	
Computer Supplies/Software	1500	4,950

TRAVEL

Patient-related 4500; Conferences 1500	6,000

PATIENT CARE COSTS	INPATIENT	
	OUTPATIENT	

ALTERATIONS AND RENOVATIONS *(Itemize by category)*

OTHER EXPENSES *(Itemize by category)*

For detailed Oth. Exp. please see page 5.	44,450

SUBTOTAL DIRECT COSTS FOR INITIAL BUDGET PERIOD

CONSORTIUM/CONTRACTUAL COSTS

DIRECT COSTS	$ 61,326	TOTAL ⟶	
INDIRECT COSTS	$ 33,729		95,055

TOTAL DIRECT COSTS FOR INITIAL BUDGET PERIOD *(Item 7a, Face Page)* ⟶ | $ 443,620 |

PERSONNEL: FIRST TWELVE MONTHS

NAME:[1]	ROLE IN PROJECT	1 TYPE APPT.	2 % EFF'T ON PROJ.	3 INST. BASE SAL.	SALARY	FRINGE	TOTALS
	RSII/Proj. Director	12	40	42,675	17,070	4,097	21,167
	RSI/Nurse Examiner	12	100	33,031	33,031	7,927	40,958
	PrinSteno/Followup Coor.	12	100	26,676	26,676	6,402	33,078
	Res Asst IV/Admin Asst	12	100	20,247	20,247	4,859	25,106
	RSII/Psychologist	5	40	42,045	16,818	4,036	20,854
	RSIV/Psychologist	4	35	49,040	17,164	4,119	21,283
	Prog/Analyst II	11	95	35,693	33,909	8,138	42,047
	Record Abstractor	6	50	24,024	12,012	2,883	14,895
TBN	Res Asst IV	12	100	18,972	18,972	4,553	23,525
TBN	Res Asst IV	6	50	18,342	9,171	2,201	11,372
TBN	Jr. Admin Asst/Sec	12	100	25,024	25,024	6,006	31,030
			TOTALS		230,094	55,221	285,315

OTHER EXPENSES (from: form page 4)
Itemized by category

Statistical Services	14,900	Patient Transp. Reimb.	1,500
Computer Usage	5,000	Medical Records	750
PC Maintenance	500	Office Rental	1,200
Audiometry	4,800	Postage	2,000
		Telephone	4,000
Specialists' Exams	7,300		
Photocopying	2,500		

TOTAL   -   44,450

---

[1] Editors' note: The names of key personnel would be given here; TBN (to be named) is indicated for persons who would be hired if the grant was supported.

EE   Principal Investigator/Program Director *(Last, first, middle)*:

BUDGET FOR ENTIRE PROPOSED PROJECT PERIOD
DIRECT COSTS ONLY

BUDGET CATEGORY TOTALS		INITIAL BUDGET PERIOD *(from page 4)*	ADDITIONAL YEARS OF SUPPORT REQUESTED			
			2nd	3rd	4th	5th
PERSONNEL: *Salary and fringe benefits* Applicant organization only		285,315	214,350			
CONSULTANT COSTS		2,300	2,300			
EQUIPMENT		5,550	0			
SUPPLIES		4,950	2,650			
TRAVEL		6,000	3,000			
PATIENT CARE COSTS	INPATIENT					
	OUTPATIENT					
ALTERATIONS AND RENOVATIONS						
OTHER EXPENSES		44,450	30,833			
SUBTOTAL DIRECT COSTS		348,565	253,133			
CONSORTIUM/ CONTRACTUAL COSTS		95,055	99,808			
TOTAL DIRECT COSTS		443,620	352,941			

TOTAL DIRECT COSTS FOR ENTIRE PROPOSED PROJECT PERIOD *(Item 8a)* ⟶ $ 796,561

JUSTIFICATION (Use continuation pages if necessary):

From Budget for Initial Period: Describe the specific functions of the personnel, collaborators, and consultants and identify individuals with appointments that are less than full time for a specific period of the year, including VA appointments.

For All Years: Explain and justify purchase of major equipment, unusual supplies requests, patient care costs, alterations and renovations, tuition remission, and donor/volunteer costs.

From Budget for Entire Period: Identify with an asterisk (*) on this page and justify any significant increase or decrease in any category over the initial budget period. Describe any change in effort of personnel.

For Competing Continuation Applications: Justify any significant increases or decreases in any category over the current level of support.

Budget Justification[2]

General Considerations

We note here that funding for this study has repeatedly been cut as part of general across the board reductions. The study section's description of our original budget stated: "Although the budget is high, it seems to be in keeping with the complexity of the project and the need for consortium arrangements." Nonetheless, study section removed $240,590 from our proposed budget. Subsequent annual reductions, also not aimed at any specific budgetary target, have removed a further $160,352 from this total. Thus in the five years of this project we have received $400,943 less than our projected need. The budget we propose for the first renewal year, in which almost all of the follow-up assessments will have been completed, is about the amount by which our budget was reduced. If we receive the funding we here request, our total per subject cost will amount to $2,372. For this sum, the following tasks will have been performed:

Abstraction of entire prenatal and neonatal record by trained nurse-abstractors. Average abstraction time per record was eight hours.

Obtaining three cranial ultrasounds at timed intervals including nights and weekends.

Double reading of ultrasounds by expert readers.

Personal interviews of mothers of study infants.

Complete neuropathologist services for infants who die.

Maintaining contact with families for two years after discharge.

Obtaining neurodevelopmental, hearing, vision and behavior assessments on all survivors including specialty examinations where necessary.

Entry of material into computer storage and creation of a cleaned and edited computer data file ready for analysis.

Publication and dissemination of research findings.

By any measure, this has to be considered cost efficient research. Neurodevelopmental assessment alone, in the depth performed in this research, would be costlier in many settings than our per subject cost.

Cost of Follow Up Examinations

Examinations of all members of a cohort such as ours is time consuming and difficult. A significant proportion of the follow up team expenditures are used to track, schedule and follow up patients who miss appointments.

We anticipate assessing 240 children in the first fiscal year of the budget. The personnel costs for actually performing these assessments (, all specialist examiners) amount to just under $400 per subject, a remarkably low figure for the in depth assessment we obtain. Maintenance of an office with telephone, stationery, supplies, postage and a computer amounts to approximately $52 per patient (the contribution of one of our offices by a consultant neurologist is an enormous benefit here). The expense for the team responsible for tracking and scheduling (   ) and for their expenditures for travel and for patient travel amounts to $270 per patient. Testing equipment has for the most part been purchased—new items requested add only about $11 per patient to costs. Our budget request for follow-up is based on actual costs incurred in the first 18 months of follow-up experience.

---

[2] Editors' note: Pages 221–226 in this Appendix have been formatted to match specifications for this volume. The reader should note that actual proposals must be typed on 8 1/2 × 11 paper and should not employ special fonts or formatting.

Personnel

(Note that   and   are budgeted in the University consortium)

Dr.   (40%) as Principal Investigator, will provide the overall scientific direction for the project, as he has for the past four years. He will ensure that a timetable for the evaluation of the study subjects and for the analysis of data is adhered to. He will direct research meetings, meet regularly with other principals and consultants, and take primary responsibility for the production of scientific papers.

Dr.   (20%) has been involved as Co principal investigator with the design and execution of this study since its inception. He attends weekly research meetings, and advises on epidemiologic issues in data collection and analysis. His firm editorial hand will undoubtedly find expression in the manuscripts we expect to be producing in the next two years.

Ms.   (10%) is the administrator of the   Center. She will oversee the budget, including the specific expenditures, and take responsibility for financial reporting. She will also supervise personnel hiring and management.

Dr.   (40%) will serve as the Project Director for the study. Dr.   has served in this capacity for the past four years. Her role is to supervise the follow-up data collection and ensure its reliability. She will continue to work closely with Mr.   in data management. She will participate in the analysis of data, and in the authorship of manuscripts.

Ms.   (100%) will act as the follow up nurse and will perform the hearing, vision and neurological screening examinations on all study subjects. These exams generally take about an hour to do. Ms.   underwent extensive training in this capacity as part of the Neonatal Brain Hemorrhage study and the reliability of her examinations has been outstanding to date (see text).

Ms.   (100%) will act as the administrative coordinator for the follow-up office. This job requires maintaining ongoing contact with the entire cohort of subjects to be seen at age two, the scheduling of the examinations, the entry of the collected follow-up data onto computer, and the disbursal of the results of the examinations to local physicians. It was only upon assigning a full-time person to this position that we began to achieve the good follow up rates reported in the text.

Ms.   (100%) joined the follow-up team last year and serves two roles. She assists Ms.   in the performance of examinations (both the hearing and vision screening requires two testers), and she assists Ms.   in contacting mothers to schedule appointments. Her addition to the follow-up team has streamlined the activities of the team and allowed them to see more subjects/week. When necessary, she also administers the health history interview and the Achenbach child behavior checklist.

                (40%)   (35%) These two part-time psychologists, both with extensive experience in infant testing, share responsibility for performing and scoring the Bayley and Zimmerman scales on our study subjects, and the Stanford-Binet examination when the infant is over 30 months (gestational-age corrected). Cognitive testing at this age takes 45–90 minutes.

Ms.   (50%) is a registered nurse who has abstracted neonatal records at the   Medical Center site. She now abstracts the medical records of followed-up infants covering the period from birth to age two years.

Mr.   (100%) will act as the chief computer programmer for the study. Mr.   has had extensive experience working with large data sets and is facile with analytic work on both microcomputers and the University mainframe. He has developed the programs for neonatal data entry and editing in this project, and will play a critical role in facilitating the analysis of the already collected data. He has begun to develop similar programs for the entry and editing of the follow-up data.

Research Assistants

1 full time and 1 half-time research assistant will work directly on Data management. This includes entry of the following data into computer storage, and working under Dr.   supervision to check data as it comes into the central office. They will also assist Mr.   exerting computer analyses under his direction.

Secretary

(100%) A full time secretary/receptionist is needed to handle the extensive communications between work in NJ and NY, and to type manuscripts emerging from the research.

Consultation Costs

Audition

Ph.D., of the   College of Medicine, will continue to work with us in maintaining our standard of audiometry and tympanometry. She will visit our field site twice, and participate in two research meetings to review and discuss data for publication. We have budgeted consulting fees for two 2-hour and two 4-hour sessions (12 hours at $25/hour=$300).

Vision

Dr.   of the University   will continue to serve as our consultant on vision screening. She will visit twice for a full 8-hour day combining a field visit with a research planning session each time (16 hours at $25/hour = $400).

Psychology

Dr.   will make three visits to the field to monitor the performance of the cognitive testing procedures and perform interrater reliability (4 hour/visit) and hold six meetings (two hours each) with the principal investigator and project director in New York City.

Travel

Reimbursement of travel expenses for consultants is estimated at $1,000. The major expense is for Dr.   , who must fly in from Pittsburgh.

Equipment

Two pieces of equipment will need replacement in the course of the study, the Teller Acuity cards ($1,050) and the tympanometer ($2,500). We anticipate that the remaining major item, the pure-tone amplifier, will last the duration of the testing period, although replacement parts are needed (see below).

PC Hardware

There is a need to replace the computer in the New Jersey follow-up office. This computer was originally used for low-level data entry. It has become the hub of scheduling and tracking the participants in the study. Additionally, the machine has become used for intensive data entry.

The research personnel are spending a significant part of the time at the computer waiting for it to accomplish searches, sorts and generate reports. This situation has inhibited personnel from performing other job responsibilities. The replacement of the machine with an AT class machine would almost eliminate this wait and allow personnel to better fulfill their job requirements.

We plan to purchase a Leading Edge model D2 80286 PC AT-compatible computer with 640K of memory, a 30 megabyte hard drive, a 1.2 floppy diskette, parallel and serial ports, a clock calendar, a monitor and monitor card. There are other manufacturers that provide a similar package: Epson, NEC, AST Research, and Hertz. The differences would be more memory and/or hard disk storage. By careful shopping in the New York area, we can obtain one Leading Edge or a very similar model for $2,000.

Supplies:

General office supplies will be needed for both the central office in New York as well as two field offices in New Jersey. Supplies for New York City will be contributed by   Center. Supplies for the two testing offices in New

Jersey amount to $2,800. This is based on actual expenses for the past fiscal year and includes stationery, pens, local copying, small office equipment, and snacks for study subjects.

Follow-up testing supplies will be purchased at an estimated cost of $650. This includes $500 for replacement parts for of audiometric equipment, and $150 for tympanometry supplies (paper, ear tips, etc.)

PC Software Purchases will amount to $1,000. We are currently spending $175 annually for a Software Maintenance Plan (SMP) for R:BASE, the data base program used to manage out data, for reduced price upgrades, telephone support, and a newsletter subscription for R:BASE. We will need to upgrade a variety of statistical programs: SPSS, SAS, 7 BMOP, at a cost of $500. We will need $325 for the purchase of new programs, i.e., plotting programs, graphics for slides, etc.

Computer Supplies are budgeted at $500. Floppy diskettes will cost $200 for 100 floppy diskettes at $2 each. Cleaning supplies for monitors, disk drives, etc. will cost approximately $100. Printer ribbons will cost $100. Computer Paper will cost $100.

Travel:

$1,500 is requested to partially cover the cost of sending Drs.   and   to the meeting of the Society for Epidemiologic Research in order to present ongoing research findings and to consult with others about their work. We also request $4,500 for local travel. This money will be used to enable the follow-up team to travel to the homes of those study subjects who refuse or are unable to make the trip to our clinic site for their two year examination. Based on past experience we anticipate that 30% of all subjects will fall into this category. The estimate of costs is based on actual cost from the most recent year. Although most trips are within a 25 mile radius, the team has driven to Pennsylvania, New York State and New Jersey to examine subjects.

Consortium/Contractual Costs:

A   University Consortium will be arranged to cover a portion of the salaries of Drs.   and Ms.   The salaries are listed in the attached Consortium budget, and are justified above.

Other Expenses

Statistical Services

The Division of Biostatistics of   University will provide statistical services. Dr.   , head of the division, will assign Dr.   to manage the statistical aspects of the projects. He will attend our weekly research meetings and assist us in the analysis of the reliability and validity of data collected as well as in the etiologic analyses to be performed.

Computer Costs:

Mainframe Analyses—$5,000

Our estimates of mainframe costs are based on a comparison to our work on New York City vital data between 1978–1984. Mainframe costs for that research were between $10,000 and $15,000 annually. The New York City data sets were a combination of vital statistics tapes from the years 1978–1984 and condensed count data sets. The total N of cases were approximately 300,000 and the total N of variables was 150. The bulk of analyses were done on the LBW data set of 13,000. Our present data set has a sample size of 1,105, and the ultrasound data set has an N of 5,560. The total N of variables for each subject is around 4,000. The cost estimate is based on the assumption that we will be able to do much of the preliminary analysis on the microcomputer. Most of these analyses would be of a descriptive type, but some of the analysis would be multivariate in nature. Intensive multivariate analyses on the mainframe will be done only on a restricted set of variables, selected following these preliminary analyses.

Computer Maintenance—$500
Five hundred dollars is requested to pay for maintenance of the equipment used for the project in New York City. Much of the equipment is five years old and approaching the mean time to breakdown.

Specialist Examination

Audiology All subjects who screen positive on the hearing portion of our two year screening examination are referred on to a pediatric ophthalmologist for more detailed testing. We anticipate approximately 20% of our 240 subjects in year 01 will require such specialized examination at a cost of $100 per patient. The audiology laboratories at   Medical Center and at Medical Center are used as referral sites ($4,800).

Neurology   , Chief of Pediatrics at the   Medical Center–Medical School will serve as our principal neurology consultant, who, along with three other child neurologists,   and   , are the final diagnosticians for all study subjects screened as neurologically abnormal or suspect by our research nurse examiner. We anticipate that about 15% of the 240 first year subjects will be referred to the neurologists, who will therefore examine approximately 36 patients in the 15 months. At a cost of $75 per patient, the budget for these examinations is $2,700. Additionally, 2 two-hour meetings to discuss neurologic findings and to review data for publication are budgeted in year 01, with each neurologist's time reimbursed at $25 per hour ($400).

Ophthalmology
Ophthalmology testing by Dr.   , our consultant pediatric ophthalmologist will be necessary for those study subjects who screen positive on our vision and eye evaluation done at the two year visit. We anticipate that approximately 10% of subjects will fall into this category. Assuming 240 subjects are seen between April 1989 and 1990, this will result in 24 vision exams at an estimated cost of $50 per exam ($1,200).

Radiology
Drs.   and   are needed to read the final 10–15% of ultrasound films not double read, and to assist in reconciling divergent readings. We estimate 60 hours work for each consultant at $25/hour ($3,000). Costs for these four groups of specialist examinations thus total $7,300.

Medical Records
Many physicians and hospitals charge for copying and forwarding medical records of study subjects. This cost is estimated at $750.00.

Office Rental
We are charged a fee of $100 per month as rent for the office space used by one of our two follow-up clinic sites, in New Jersey. The site in Neptune, New Jersey is part of Dr.   office suite, and generously contributed by her.

Postage
A large volume of material is mailed out by our follow-up office, including follow-up letters at six month intervals after discharge to keep in contact with the families, a letter to invite the subject to participate in the two-year examination, a set of forms to be filled out by the mother prior to her child's two year examination, a request to the pediatrician for the medical records of the child from birth to two years of age, the results of the two year examination to inform the pediatrician of the child's performance, thank you letters and other miscellaneous items. This volume of material will require a postage budget of $2,000.

Telephone

Tracking down the study subjects two years after discharge from the hospital necessitates a large volume of long distance telephone calling. Based on our current experience, we estimate our telephone expenses for both the central office in New York and the follow-up office in New Jersey to be $3,000.

Transportation Reimbursement

Some of our study subjects, who will be willing to attend our follow-up clinic, will be without their own transportation. In such a situation, we will offer to cover the cost of transportation to and from the clinic in order to increase attendance. We anticipate that approximately 50 subjects will require such an incentive at a cost of approximately $30 per subject ($1,500).

Copying

A large volume of copying of forms, letters, and computer printouts and articles, take place both at the study site and the NY office. Our estimated cost is $2,500.

YEAR 2

The budget for year 2 is based on the following assumptions: 320 children need to be seen, of whom 240 will be seen in the first year, leaving 80 in year 2, to be seen over approximately 4 months. The personnel involved in follow-up are thus budgeted for 40% salaries, allowing a few weeks extra to examine late stragglers. Equipment costs will be nil, and New Jersey supplies, patient costs, telephone, postage, and travel are also budgeted at one-third of the first year expenditure. The members of the data analysis team are maintained at the same rate as Year 1 as are the three consultants, who will be involved in data analysis. Computer costs (excluding the computer purchase) are maintained as in year 1. All salaries are increased 5% to account for inflation.

DD

Principal Investigator/Program Director *(Last, first, middle):* _____

University Consortium

DETAILED BUDGET FOR INITIAL BUDGET PERIOD **DIRECT COSTS ONLY**	FROM 04/01/89	THROUGH 03/31/90

PERSONNEL *(Applicant organization only)*		TYPE APPT. *(months)*	% EFFORT ON PROJ.	INST. BASE SALARY	DOLLAR AMOUNT REQUESTED *(omit cents)*		
NAME	ROLE ON PROJECT				SALARY REQUESTED	FRINGE BENEFITS	TOTALS
	Principal Investigator				33,933	9,162	43,095
	Co-Investig.	12	10	106,230	10,623	2,868	13,491
	Admin. Coord.	12	10	37,320	3,732	1,008	4,740
SUBTOTALS →					48,288	13,038	61,326

CONSULTANT COSTS	
EQUIPMENT *(Itemize)*	
SUPPLIES *(Itemize by category)*	
TRAVEL	

PATIENT CARE COSTS	INPATIENT	
	OUTPATIENT	

ALTERATIONS AND RENOVATIONS *(Itemize by category)*	

OTHER EXPENSES *(Itemize by category)* Indirect Cost – 55% of MTDC	33,729	33,729

SUBTOTAL DIRECT COSTS FOR INITIAL BUDGET PERIOD	95,055

CONSORTIUM/CONTRACTUAL COSTS		
DIRECT COSTS $	TOTAL →	
INDIRECT COSTS $		

TOTAL DIRECT COSTS FOR INITIAL BUDGET PERIOD *(Item 7a, Face Page)* →	$	95,055

228

EE

Principal Investigator/Program Director *(Last, first, middle):* _____

University
Consortium

**BUDGET FOR ENTIRE PROPOSED PROJECT PERIOD
DIRECT COSTS ONLY**

BUDGET CATEGORY TOTALS		INITIAL BUDGET PERIOD *(from page 4)*	ADDITIONAL YEARS OF SUPPORT REQUESTED			
			2nd	3rd	4th	5th
PERSONNEL: *Salary and fringe benefits* Applicant organization only		61,326	64,392			
CONSULTANT COSTS						
EQUIPMENT						
SUPPLIES						
TRAVEL						
PATIENT CARE COSTS	INPATIENT					
	OUTPATIENT					
ALTERATIONS AND RENOVATIONS						
OTHER EXPENSES		33,729	35,416			
SUBTOTAL DIRECT COSTS		95,055	99,808			
CONSORTIUM/ CONTRACTUAL COSTS						
TOTAL DIRECT COSTS		95,055	99,808			

TOTAL DIRECT COSTS FOR ENTIRE PROPOSED PROJECT PERIOD *(Item 8a)* ⟶ $ 194,863

JUSTIFICATION (Use continuation pages if necessary):

From Budget for Initial Period: Describe the specific functions of the personnel, collaborators, and consultants and identify individuals with appointments that are less than full time for a specific period of the year, including VA appointments.

For All Years: Explain and justify purchase of major equipment, unusual supplies requests, patient care costs, alterations and renovations, tuition remission, and donor/volunteer costs.

From Budget for Entire Period: Identify with an asterisk (*) on this page and justify any significant increase or decrease in any category over the initial budget period. Describe any change in effort of personnel.

For Competing Continuation Applications: Justify any significant increases or decreases in any category over the current level of support.

Salary rates have been increased 5% annually. Fringe rate remains at 27% throughout.

Appendix C
Charts, Timelines, and Other Visual Aids

Budget Justification[1]

We begin this budget justification by calling the readers' attention to the figures immediately following this page. These figures provide information in graphic form on sampling, sample sizes, sequencing of evaluation procedures, subject flow from one procedure to the next, and criteria for selection into the different evaluations. The text of the budget justification provides additional information on the rationale and practical details of these aspects of the proposed study. We have provided the visual information separately for male and female subjects in addition to presenting the information for the combined total sample, since the "yield" (the proportions expected to be positive on the different measures) will differ for males and females. This information responds to the reviewers' well-taken critiques of our original submission that the description of these aspects of the study was unclear and needed to be better developed.

Figure 3 and Insets 3a, 3b, and 3c provide corresponding information for the total sample, combining males and females. Figure 4 illustrates how the required numbers of interviews will be distributed chronologically over the time of the study. Figure 5 illustrates the staff organizational structure of the study.

Throughout, we have based sample size requirements on considerations of adequate statistical power for the analyses we have planned. The expected "yields" (proportions positive from the different procedures) were determined from analyses of data from the 1984 national survey of the drinking practices and problems of adults conducted by the Alcohol Research Group, an MIAAA research center. This sample of 5221 adults, selected according to standard practices for drawing a national sample from which nationally representative rates can be derived, allowed computation of rates of alcohol use disorders, subclinical manifestations of alcohol problems, and heavy drinking in the U.S. general population.

To clarify a point that evidently was quite unclear in the original submission of this grant, note that the initial brief screen, which will take only a few minutes to administer, is NOT designed to positively identify subjects with alcohol abuse or dependence, but to identify those with a greatly increased probability of having these disorders, compared to the general population. This brief screen is used in order to make the study possible without requiring a greatly increased budget. Subjects passing this brief screen are considered "included" in the study and are evaluated more extensively.

The reviewers of the original grant raised a well-taken point about differential effects of telephone vs.

[1] Editors' note: Pages 229, 231, 233, and 235–242 in this Appendix have been formatted to match specifications for this volume. The reader should note that actual proposals must be typed on 8 1/2 × 11 paper and should not employ special fonts or formatting.

Preliminary screen
(phone or at-home)
N = 5950
screen positive*
N=1875
screen negative*
N=4075 ->no further contact
ADQ interview
(in person)
N = 1875
Alcohol Dependent
All other categories
N=50
N=50
ADQ reliability study
ALCOHOL DEPENDENT
N = 260
Alcohol abuse
N=180
Abuse/dep. negative
N=1335
>sub-group split
sub-clinical
N=280
consecutive negatives
N=280
remaining negatives
N=775
no further contact
SCID interview
(in person)
N = 1000
all
LIFE-A interview
(in person, 1 year later)
N = 1000
N=50
N=50
LIFE-A reliability retest
clinical re-interview
Inset 1a
Inset 1b
Inset 1c
Inset 1d

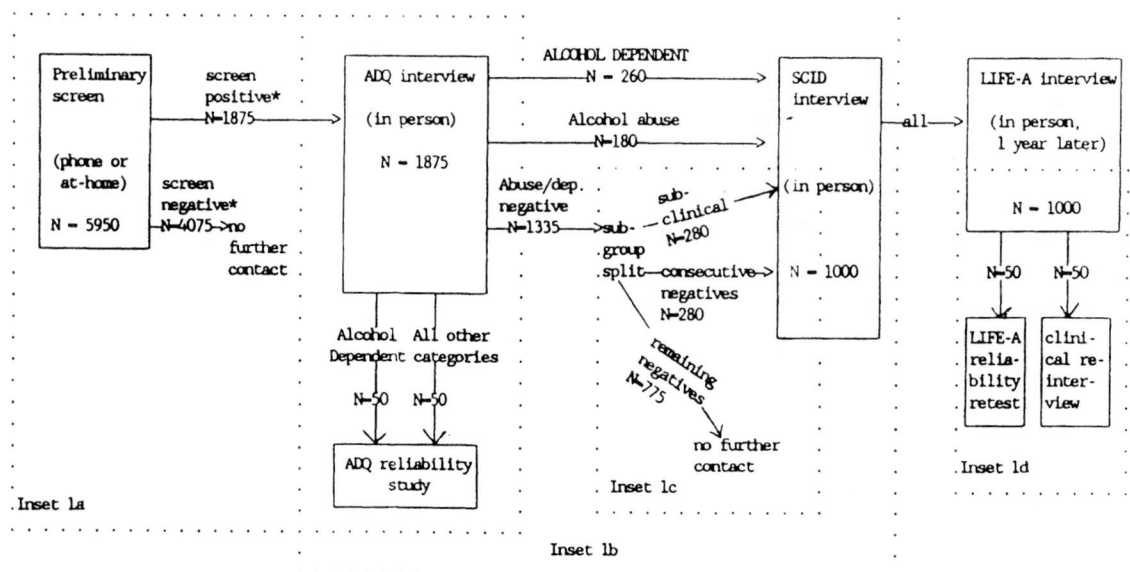

Figure 3. Interview sequence for all subjects (males and females combined). Screen positive = 5 or more drinks on a single occasion in the last year. Screen negative = no such drinking occasions in last year.

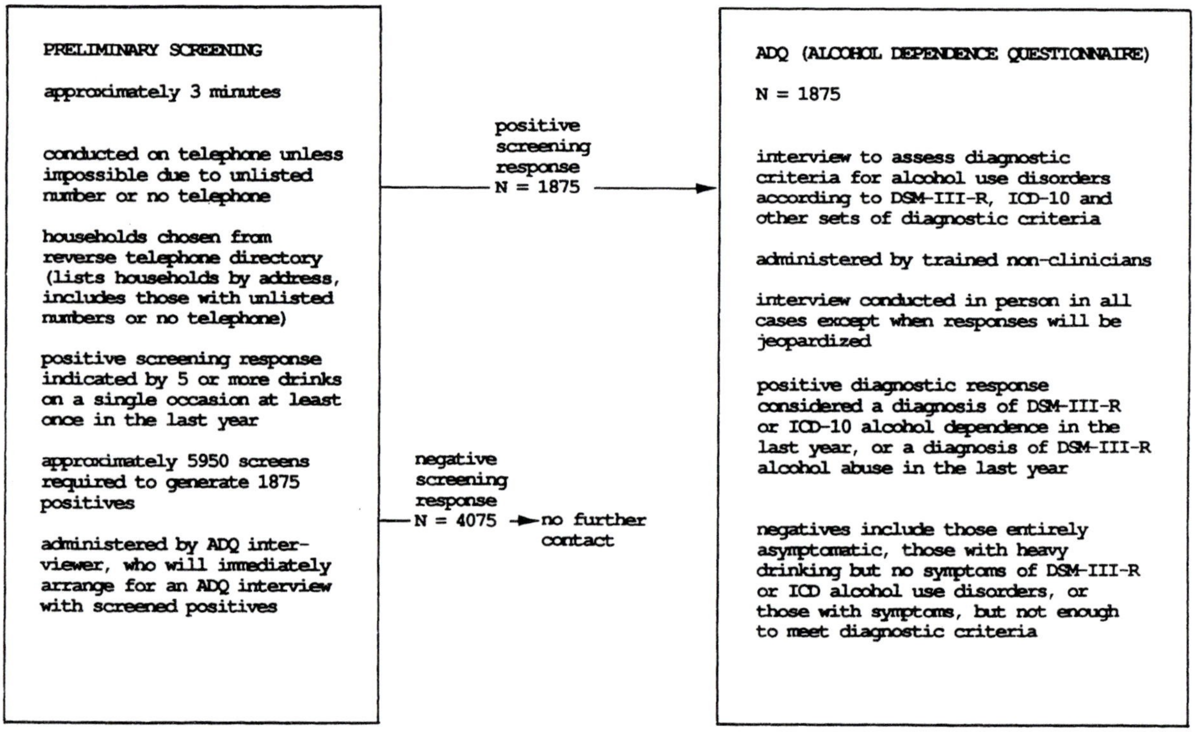

PRELIMINARY SCREENING
approximately 3 minutes
conducted on telephone unless impossible due to unlisted number or no telephone
households chosen from reverse telephone directory (lists households by address, includes those with unlisted numbers or no telephone)
positive screening response indicated by 5 or more drinks on a single occasion at least once in the last year
approximately 5950 screens required to generate 1875 positives
administered by ADQ interviewer, who will immediately arrange for an ADQ interview with screened positives
positive screening response
N = 1875
negative screening response
N = 4075
no further contact
ADQ (ALCOHOL DEPENDENCE QUESTIONNAIRE)
N = 1875
interview to assess diagnostic criteria for alcohol use disorders according to DSM-III-R, ICD-10 and other sets of diagnostic criteria
administered by trained non-clinicians
interview conducted in person in all cases except when responses will be jeopardized
positive diagnostic response considered a diagnosis of DSM-III-R or ICD-10 alcohol dependence in the last year, or a diagnosis of DSM-III-R alcohol abuse in the last year
negatives include those entirely asymptomatic, those with heavy drinking but no symptoms of DSM-III-R or ICD alcohol use disorders, or those with symptoms, but not enough to meet diagnostic criteria

Inset 3a. Sequence from preliminary screening to administration of ADQ interview, all subjects combined (males and females).

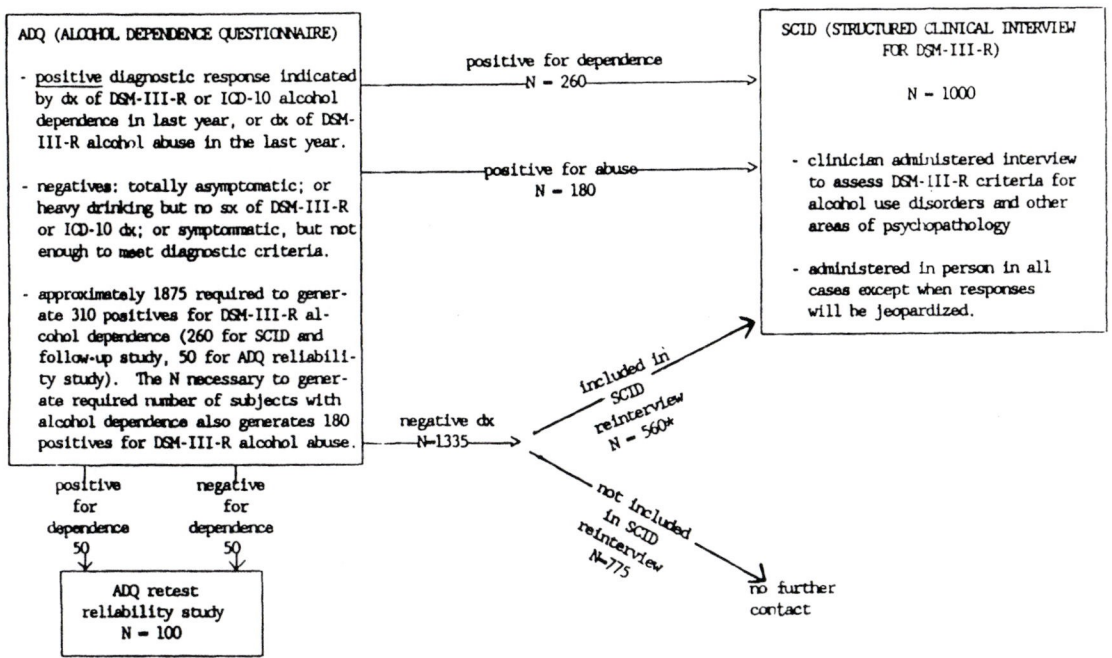

Inset 3b. Sequence from administration of ADQ interview to administration of SCID interview, all subjects (males and females combined). * = see Inset 3c for additional detail on selection at this point.

in-person evaluation. Use of the telephone as much as possible to screen (about 70% of the individuals who might potentially be included in the study) results in significant savings in the budget. Underestimates in reporting alcohol consumption and problems would preclude use of the telephone when (a) the research aim is to generate consumption rates in a given geographic area, or (b) to make a thorough evaluation of an individual's history of consumption and problems. However, a telephone screening process does not create a problem if the purpose is to cost-effectively generate a group of untreated individuals for further study who acknowledge a recent history of at least moderately high consumption. Since generation of such a group is the sole purpose of screening in this study, we have elected the telephone option for screening whenever possible to reduce costs.

In the text below, we describe and justify the costs necessary to accomplish the work outlined in the figures over the three years of requested support. Additional details on the work and personnel required for this are also described below. Costs are based on our prior experience, guidelines from and the number of anticipated evaluations done in each year. In some cases, we have chosen salary levels that will allow us to hire staff members already experienced in departmental procedures.

We note that in all aspects of the budget, we have tried to control costs without precluding the achievement of the goals of the study. The amount we have requested has increased from our last submission due primarily to modifications made in response to the reviewers' comments on the study from the first submission. These include (a) a change in design to administer all procedures except the initial screening in person, rather than allowing the option of some telephone interviewing, and (b) better development of the rationale for including subjects in the SCID clinical reinterview and the one-year follow-up interview. The clearer rationale for inclusion and exclusion of subjects in these portions of the study led to our increasing somewhat the numbers of subjects re-interviewed with the SCID and followed

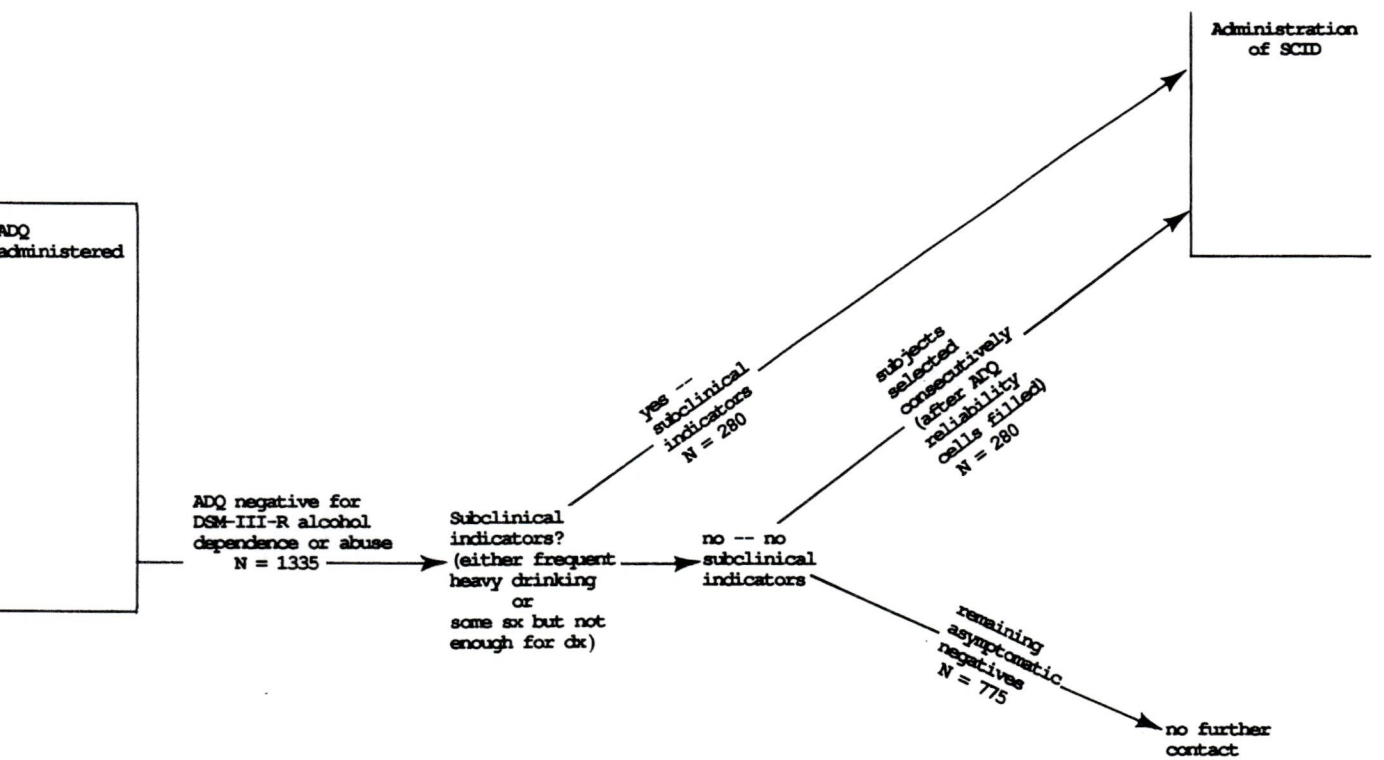

Inset 3c. Selection of subjects with no ADQ DSM-III-R alcohol abuse or dependence diagnosis into SCID reinterview study and follow up study, all subjects (males and females combined).

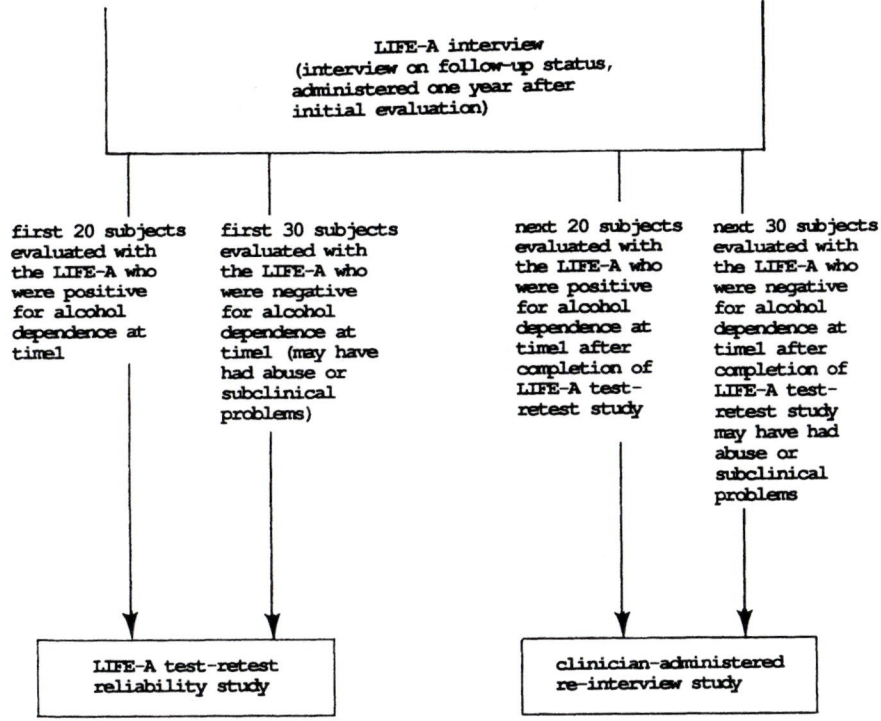

Figure 3d. Selection of subjects (males and females combined) into LIFE-A reliability study and clinician re-interview study.

up one year later. Budget increases also resulted to a small degree from cost-of-living increases in salary levels for staff.

Payment for the non-clinician interviewers is described in the section on personnel. However, on the actual budget pages themselves, this part of the budget is listed under "other expenses". We have listed the non-clinician payment this way due to administrative procedures for paying such raters by the interview on a contract basis rather than having them on salary.

Year 01

Personnel: Core Staff

Principal Investigator (50% Time, Salary Contributed for Year 01) Dr.   , the PI, will be responsible for overall organization and management of the project, in conjunction with the Co-PI, Dr.   . She will hire and train clinical and non-clinical raters and supervise the protocol monitor. Dr.   will share supervision of raters with the protocol monitor, see below. This will include periodic monitoring of interviewing by listening to audiotapes of interviews conducted in the field, as well as periodic training updates and personnel issues. Dr.   will supervise data entering as well as cleaning, both pre- and post-entry. In the early stages of the study, Dr.   will do some interviewing of both types with subjects to identify practical problems with the procedures and to provide familiarity that

```
1990                              1991                         1992
Ap My Jn Jl Ag St Ot Nv Dc Jn Fb Mr Ap My Jn Jl Ag St Ot Nv Dc Jn Fb Mr Ap My Jn Jl Ag St Ot Nv Dc Jn Fb Mr

Start-
Up
        ——— At-home screens (140/month) ———>  55 50 †

        ——————— ADQs (150/month*) ————————>  50 25 †

        ——————— SCIDs (80/month**) ———————>  20 20 †

     ==>                            ——————— Follow-ups (85/month***) ———> 40 40 †
  Reliability                         ==>
 analyses, write-up                Reliability
      (ADQ)                       analyses, write-up
                                      (LIFE-A)
                                       ===== Cross-sect'l/concrdnce ======>
                                            analyses, write-ups
                                                           ==== Follow-up ===>
                                                           analyses, write-ups
```

*   includes 100 additional by the end of July, 1990, to complete the ADQ reliability retest interviews

**   plus 50 additional by the end of July, 1990, to complete the SCID reliability retest interviews

*** includes 100 additional by the end of June, 1991, to complete the LIFE-A reliability and clinical reinterview studies

†   freestanding numbers to the right of arrows indicate the numbers of interviews to be conducted during the months indicated directly above the freestanding number.

Figure 4. Time line.

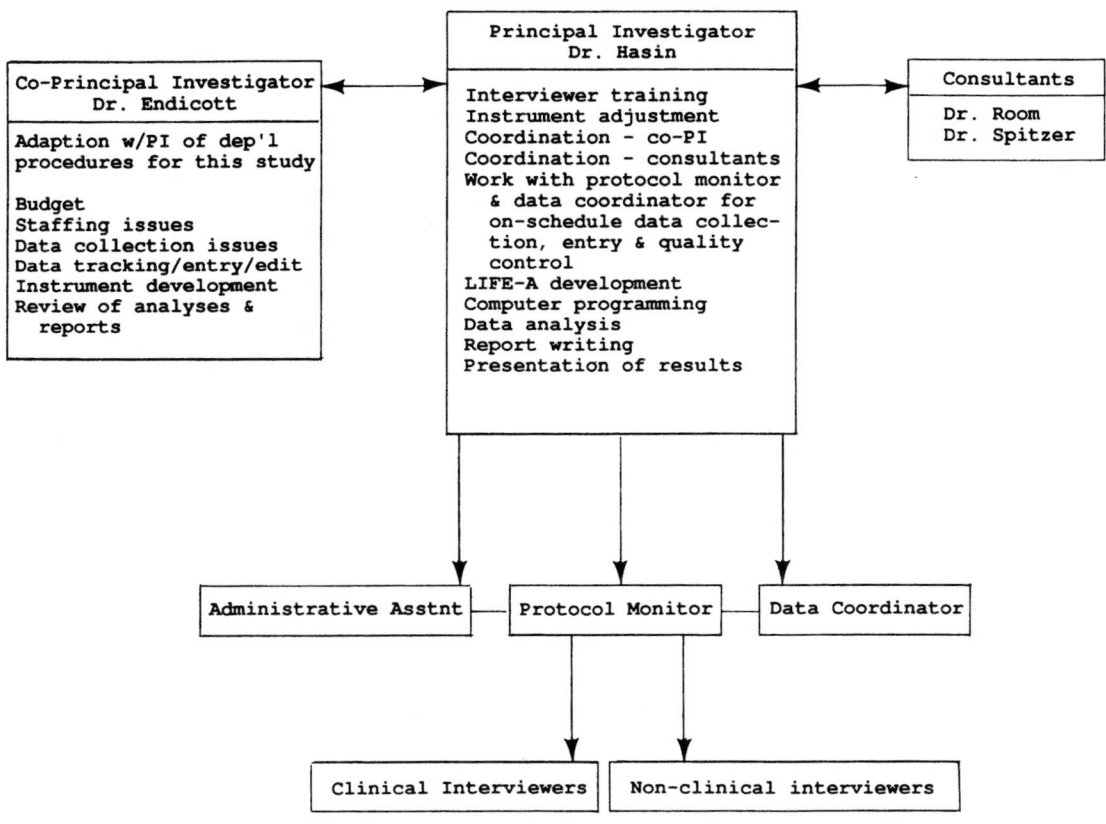

Figure 5. Organizational chart.

will enhance later interpretation of the results. Dr.⠀⠀⠀⠀will perform all computer programming and data analyses once the data is clean. (Her training and experience with biostatistics and the computer enables her to do this and saves the cost of an additional staff member to perform these functions.) She will take primary responsibility for the preparation of reports, articles, and presentations, collaborating with Dr. ⠀⠀⠀on this work. Funding is not requested for Dr.⠀⠀⠀⠀'s salary for year 01 since her salary is covered from other sources during this time.

Co-Principal Investigator (10% Time, Contributed) Since the center for scientific, administrative and data processing aspects of the study will be located in Dr.⠀⠀⠀⠀'s department at ⠀⠀⠀. Dr.⠀⠀⠀, the co-PI, will work with Dr.⠀⠀⠀⠀on adapting departmental procedures used successfully in the past to take into account the needs of the proposed study. This will include budget issues, the relationship of aspects of the study in the department to the institute as a whole, rater hiring, training, and supervision, subject recruitment and scheduling, tracking of data, data entry and editing. Also, in conjunction with Dr.⠀⠀⠀, Dr.⠀⠀⠀will coordinate the project with the other research taking place in the department. Dr.⠀⠀⠀will confer with Dr.⠀⠀⠀in resolving problems encountered in recruiting subjects and retaining them in the study.

Dr.⠀⠀⠀will work with Dr.⠀⠀⠀on the development of measures and scales. Dr.⠀⠀⠀will also review all reliability, concordance and validity data as it is assembled, advising Dr.⠀⠀⠀of her interpretation of the material on an ongoing basis. In addition, Dr.　　　will assist in the preparation of reports and articles, and carefully review all written material as it is completed. Funding is not requested for Dr.　　's time because she has full support.

Protocol Monitor (100%) The protocol monitor will assume primary responsibility for administration of subject recruiting and interviewing. He or she will monitor respondent "compliance" and supervise interviewers in terms of completing the necessary number of interviews per week. The protocol monitor will monitor interviewing quality, and act as an interface between the data coordinator (see below) and interviewers to ensure completeness and accuracy of coding. He/she will work with interviewers to obtain participation from unwilling or difficult-to-contact respondents. The protocol monitor will provide continued reliability information on the interviewers by periodically using audiotapes of interviews conducted in the field to blindly rate subjects' responses. These ratings will be compared to the interviewers' ratings to ensure that responses are being scored consistently and correctly. Listening to the audiotapes will also provide information to the protocol monitor on whether the interviewers are continuing to administer the interview correctly. If interviewers begin to deviate from correct procedures, this will be apparent in the audiotapes and the protocol monitor will work with the interviewers to correct any problems. The protocol monitor will also periodically but regularly contact a small number of interviewed subjects to confirm that they have, in fact, actually been interviewed and to verify some of their responses with them. The protocol monitor will also compute completion statistics, and assist with the preparation of reports as needed.

Administrative Assistant (100%) Correspondence, word processing, preparation and mailing of study announcements, telephone screening for any respondents who call in and others as needed. Payment of subject fees and travel costs. Ordering supplies, handling payroll issues, timesheets and other grant records, assist the PI in management of funds. Assisting with other activities, such as library research, as needed.

Data Editor/Coordinator (100%)
Logging in and checking interviews for completeness and accuracy prior to keypunch entry. Keypunching (or screen entry, as applicable). Working with principal investigator on monitoring quality of data and on data cleaning post-entry. Assisting with other activities such as preparing summary tables, assisting with preparation of reports.

Non-clinician Interviewers

Number of ADQ Interviews Required Our computations of the number of interviews required from our analyses are based on our analyses of the 1984 national survey data on drinking practices and problems mentioned above. This data is the most complete and current source of information available on expected frequencies of cases of DSM-III-R alcohol dependence, abuse, subclinical alcohol problems, asymptomatic heavy drinking, and the absence of these conditions. We expect that this source of data provides approximations only. We have generally rounded numbers in the conservative direction to compensate for possible attrition.

As described in the statistical analysis portion of the validity section, we need to recruit a sample of subjects in which approximately 130 males and 130 females receive a diagnosis of DSM-III-R alcohol dependence within the year prior to the interview. We also need approximately 25 male and 25 female subjects positive for alcohol dependence for the ADQ reliability study. ARG 1984 data showed that about 19% of males who have had at least five drinks on an occasion at least once in the past year received such a diagnosis. The 1984 survey data also showed that about 15% of females who had had at least five drinks on an occasion in the last year met criteria for alcohol dependence in the previous year. Given this information, we have used the 5+ drinks on an occasion experience as a simple screening device to increase the yield of alcohol use disorders in the sample of subjects interviewed with the ADQ.

The screening questions on alcohol consumption are included in a very brief set of questions which can be administered over the telephone (see description in the methods section and a copy of the questions in the appendix) to approximately 70% of the number of community residents required to yield the informative number of ADQ interviews. The ADQ interviewers will administer the screen, providing greater continuity between completion of screening and completion of the ADQ interviews. Therefore, most of the cost of this preliminary screening is considered to be covered in the payment made to the ADQ interviewers for completed interviews (see below for additional description of brief screens which must be administered in person).

After screening for a history of consumption of at least five drinks at least once in the past year, we will need to conduct approximately 775 ADQ interviews with males screened positive in order to identify the required number with the alcohol dependence diagnosis. We will also need ADQ interviews with approximately 1100 females to identify the required number of positive females (total, 1875 ADQ interviews). Establishing a sample with an informative number of female subjects adds to the cost of the project, but such a plan has seldom been carried out, resulting in a near-total lack of knowledge about validity issues concerning alcohol dependence as related to women.

We note that the interviews conducted with subjects who do not meet criteria for alcohol dependence are not wasted. Based on our analyses of the 1984 national survey, we expect that approximately 180 subjects (90 males and 90 females) who do not meet criteria for DSM-III-R alcohol dependence will meet criteria for DSM-III-R alcohol abuse. In addition, approximately 20% of the subjects who do not meet criteria for alcohol abuse or dependence will have either subclinical manifestations of alcohol problems, or frequent, heavy drinking which is asymptomatic. Identification of these subjects is important both for comparative purposes in analyses of alcohol dependence, and also as high-risk groups for studying predictors of the onset and offset of alcohol use disorders. In addition, some subjects without any alcohol problems are necessary for comparison purposes in the analyses.

ADQ Non-clinician Interviewers There are many social work, psychology and other health-related graduate programs in the area. Therefore, we anticipate that most non-clinical interviewing will be done by graduate students and other interviewers with at least bachelor's degrees. Non-clinician interviewers will be paid by the interview, as this substantially reduces personnel costs and provides staff flexibility. Contract arrangements will be made with the interviewers for payment as the work is completed.

Amount Requested During Year 01 to Pay ADQ Interviewers We have based the amount of our payment per interview on our experience and the experience of other researchers in the medical center. We will pay interviewers $80 per interview. This rate of pay takes into account the fact that between one and three brief telephone screening interviews will need to be done for each actual interview, in addition to coding, checking, and going over any interviews with core staff.

In order to generate the required number of subjects positive for DSM-III-R alcohol dependence, we will need to conduct 1875 ADQ interviews. Thus, the interviewer costs for this part of the study total $150,000. Note that while we have planned to complete most of the initial interviews during the first year, some will be completed in the second year. As shown in Figure 4, we expect to conduct an average of approximately 150 ADQ interviews a month from May to the end of the following February, with 100 additional ADQ interviews for the ADQ reliability study early in the study. Thus, for the first year, we have requested $128,000 to pay the ADQ interviewers.

An additional expense arises in this portion of the study due to the fact that about thirty percent of the residents of suburban Essex County (the county in which the proposed study will take place) do not have listed telephone numbers, either because they are unlisted or the household has no phone. Therefore, the brief screening process will require in-person visits to households for these subjects. Many of the households will be located quite close together geographically (in terms of car travel time), and an interviewer could potentially complete three or four screens in one outing (if none of these screens identifies a respondent who will be invited to participate in a full interview and who agrees to do the interview at that time). Given the extra travel time required to conduct the in-person screens, interviewers will be paid separately for conducting the screens. We request funds to pay them $25 per completed in-person screening interview. We anticipate that an average of approximately 140 home screens per month will be conducted, with a total of 1400 during the first year. Therefore, we have requested $35,000 to pay the ADQ interviewers for conducting these screening interviews.

We expect to hire approximately 15 ADQ interviewers over the course of the study. We anticipate that training the ADQ interviewers will take about 20 hours. If interviewers are paid $10/hour for training, we will need $3000 to pay for interviewer training.

3,000	interviewer training
128,000	interviewer payment for 1600 ADQ interviews
35,000	preliminary screens done in person rather than on the phone
$166,000	total cost for ADQ non-clinician interviews

We have elected to keep the data collection work in-house, rather than contract it out to a survey firm. We have done so for a number of reasons. We have wished to keep costs in this location as low as possible. More important, however, we wish to stay in closer touch with the assessment and data collection procedures than would be possible if another group were responsible for collecting the data. The focus of the grant is on assessment issues, and our experience and expertise in the development and use of measures such as those proposed for this study are unlikely to be matched by non-specialists. We note that during the study, we will have refined out procedures and developed a great deal of training materials (written manuals, videotapes, case vignettes, etc.). By the end of the study, these should be usable by others for both large and smaller-scale research projects.

Clinician Interviewers

As described in the grant, we will require interviewers with clinical training and experience to conduct SCID interviews. Psychiatrists, psychologists and psychiatric social workers usually have the training and experience to conduct SCID interviews. There are many qualified individuals in this area to do SCID interviewing, including clinicians who are already familiar with the SCID. (Some have already expressed interest to us in doing interviews for the study.)

Number of Interviews Required Whether or not a subject is interviewed with the SCID will depend on the results of his or her ADQ interview (see Figure 3 and accompanying insets and text of proposal). The ADQ will indicate whether subjects appear positive for DSM-III-R alcohol abuse or dependence, positive for subclinical manifestations of these problems or regular heavy drinking, or appear negative for any of these conditions. The approximate number of subjects likely to be in each cell is predicted from our analyses of data from the 1984 national survey on drinking practices and problems mentioned above.

We will conduct a SCID interview with all subjects whose ADQ interview indicates a likely diagnosis of DSM-III-R alcohol dependence, DSM-III-R alcohol abuse, with all subjects who have subthreshold alcohol problems without meeting diagnostic criteria, and with all subjects who are asymptomatic but who report drinking very heavily with some regularity (eight or more drinks at least once a week). Power requirements of the analyses do not require interviews from all remaining asymptomatic subjects, although some are required. Therefore, a consecutive series of the remaining subjects who have no alcohol disorder symptoms and who do not engage in regular heavy drinking will also be reinterviewed with the SCID.

Using computations from the 1984 data in conjunction with the needs for sufficient power in the statistical analyses, we have planned initial samples to yield approximately 260 subjects positive for alcohol dependence in the ADQ (130 males and 130 females). We expect approximately 180 additional subjects to test positive for alcohol abuse (90 males and 90 females). Additional computations show that we will have approximately 130 males and 150 females with subclinical alcohol problems or heavy drinking. We will administer the SCID interview to these subjects, as well as to the first 150 males and 130 females who are entirely negative for alcohol problems or regular heavy drinking. This is a total of 1000 SCID interviews. (Note that only a proportion of these are completed in the first year; see below.) The completion of this number of SCID interviews will provide data not only to compare systematic clinician assessment of alcohol use disorders with the ADQ, but will also provide a rich data base to investigate the impact of other psychopathology on the course of alcohol dependence, alcohol abuse, and subclinical alcohol-related conditions. Thus, the groundwork will be laid to achieve some of the long-range goals of the study.

To demonstrate reliability of the SCID for this study, we will need to conduct 50 SCID interviews and 50 SCID re-interviews with the same subjects. In order to reduce costs and complications, and also to provide SCID retest information with subjects who are not unduly fatigued from already participating in two interviews for this study, we will recruit subjects for the SCID test-retest reliability study from volunteers from around the medical center. The developers of the SCID used this method in the original SCID non-patient reliability study. They found that a sample sufficiently rich in psychopathology for a reliability study could be ascertained without extraordinary costs through this method.

Amount Requested During Year 01 to Pay SCID Interviewers A large proportion of the SCID interviewing will be conducted during the first year of requested support. As shown in Figure 4, an average of approximately 80 SCIDs will be done per month (after the initial start-up period), with the additional 100 reliability interviews (50 test, 50 retest) done by June, 1990. Thus, 900 SCIDs will be done in the first year. We will pay the clinician raters $100 an interview. The interviewer cost for the SCIDs will therefore be $90,000. SCID raters will also need training. The training will be relatively brief, since only selected sections of the SCID will be administered, and these are not the most complicated sections. We will pay SCID interviewers $400 for training. We anticipate hiring about 10 SCID raters and so will need $4000 for training, for a total of $94,000. According to RFMH guidelines and for simplification, we have budgeted and presented the cost of paying the SCID interviewers in approximate percent time of the appropriate RFMH grade level employees rather than as 10 separate interviewers. This results in amounts which approximate the figure of $94,000 rather than reproducing it exactly.

Consultants Dr.   , Scientific Director of   , has an international reputation as a leading researcher in the alcohol epidemiology field. He has had extensive experience in large-scale general population surveys of drinking practices and problems. He has served on several of the WHO committees which determined the ICD definitions of the dependence syndrome. Dr.   will be available on an as-needed basis to answer questions related to the study. Dr.   will come to New York early in the first year of the grant for a full-day meeting. After that, consultation can be carried out by telephone. Dr.   's fee is $1000 a year, and an additional $800 is budgeted for his trip the first year.

        , M.D., served as the chairperson of the task force on nomenclature for the   for many years, and had primary responsibility for organizing the numerous stages of work which resulted in DSM-III and DSM-III-R. Dr.   is thus arguably the most authoritative source on the intent and background of the diagnostic criteria for alcohol dependence. Dr.   , whose department is contiguous with the department in which the proposed study will be carried out, is available on an as-needed basis to answer questions about the diagnostic criteria and the SCID. He will also review questions designed to ascertain diagnoses of alcohol dependence by DSM-III-R criteria, a process which has already begun. He will also review reports on the findings of this study, offering his interpretations of our results. Dr.   's time on this study is contributed, since he has full support.

Supplies: General office supplies, folders, disks, labels, liftoff tapes.

Travel *In response to reviewers' comments, we have reduced our request for the costs of the PI's travel.* We are currently requesting funds for travel to one national conference, the American Public Health Association meeting in October, 1990. We have retained the request for one trip to Europe (for presentation of the study at two international alcoholism conferences which take place in consecutive weeks). We have retained this request because there is no other source of funding for travel to these conferences. We note that attendance at presentations and informal discussions at these international meetings in the past has stimulated a number of research ideas for Dr.   , has resulted in collaborative work with other researchers, and has assisted in the refinement of many of the ideas presented in this grant proposal.

Other Expenses: Subject Payment Subject payment is a large expense in this study. However, we feel that it is essential to supply motivation for subjects who otherwise would not participate in the interview(s) for the study. We will pay subjects $25 per interview (for each ADQ, SCID and reliability interview). Thus, we will need $62,500 to cover subject fees. We have also requested money for postage so that we can mail the study announcements to subjects prior to contacting them directly, and to mail payment to subjects after the interview(s) take place.

Year 02

Personnel

For the second year of the study, the time commitments of the PI and the Co-PI will remain the same as described for the first year. However, Dr.   's salary is only covered from other sources for the first four months of year 02. Therefore, we have asked for 8 months of support for the 50% of her commitment to this project, or one-third of a year's total salary. Dr.   's salary remains fully covered, and her time spent on this study is contributed during the second year.

While the total number of interviews will be less the second year, we will be completing the initial interviews (both the ADQs and SCIDs) and starting up the follow-up portion of the study. We anticipate that the follow-up study will require a great deal of administrative attention. Therefore, we have budgeted for a second year of full-time support for the administrative staff: the protocol monitor, administrative assistant and the data coordinator. The salary requests reflect performance advances in accordance with   guidelines, and a 5% cost-of-living increase for all administrative staff.

As noted above, we do not plan to complete all SCIDs in the first year. In the second year, there will be approximately 200 remaining SCIDs to complete. There will also be 50 clinical follow-up reinterviews (which will be conducted by SCID interviewers), for a total of 250 clinical interviews. Continuing to pay interviewers $100 per completed interview, this will cost $25,000. Clinician interviewer training for the follow-up procedure is expected to cost $2000.

Consultants

The participation of the consultants will remain the same during the second year, except that Dr.   will not need to come to New York.

Travel

Travel costs will remain the same during the second year.

Other Expenses: Non-Clinical Interviewers

To achieve the necessary total number of subjects in the study, we will complete the remaining 375 ADQ interviews in the second year. The interviewer costs for these will be the same per interview as the costs during the first year ($80 per interview). This results in a cost of $30,000. There will also be approximately 385 brief home screens. At $25 per home screen, interviewer costs for these will be $9625.

As discussed in the methods section, we anticipate a follow-up interview one year after participation in the initial phase of the study. We plan to include as many as possible of the 1000 subjects who received a SCID interview at time 1 in the follow-up. This will include subjects who met criteria for alcohol abuse or dependence at the first interview, those with sub-clinical alcohol problems or evidence of regular heavy drinking, and a consecutive subset of the remaining subjects without any evidence of alcohol problems or heavy drinking. Since most of the time 1 interviews will take place during year 01, most of the time 2 interviews will take place during year 02, although some will come due in year 03 (see below). The LIFE-A, the follow-up interview, will be administered by the non-clinician interviewers. We expect to complete most, but not all, of these interviews during the second year. We will keep the interviewer payment the same for the follow-up interviews, $80. We anticipate completing approximately 850 follow-up interviews during the second year of the study, for a cost in interviewer payments of $68,000. (We will attempt to obtain some informant information on subjects who are unlocateable or deceased, and thus have budgeted to pay ADQ interviewers to obtain this information for subjects who cannot be interviewed directly.) The non-clinical interviewers will need to be trained to administer the follow-up procedures. We anticipate paying the interviewers $200 for their time during this training. This adds another $3000. Therefore, the payment to the non-clinician interviewers totals as follows:

$30,000	remaining ADQs
9,625	home screens
68,000	LIFE-As (follow-up interviews)
3,000	interviewer training for the LIFE-A
$110,625	

Subject Payments

Subject payment will be the same for the follow-up as for the initial interview. At $25 per interview, $36,875 will be needed for subject payment in year 02 (375 ADQs, 250 clinical interviews, and 850 follow-ups).

Year 03

During the third year, the remainder of the follow-up data will be collected, and analyses and reports completed. We have requested salary support for the protocol monitor only for the first six months of the third year to oversee completion of the data collection. Dr.   will be analyzing the data from the initial interviews and preparing this material for presentation and publication. Once data collection is complete for the follow-up study, she will then focus on analyzing and writing up this part of the data. As was the case for years 01 and 02, we have not requested resources for a programmer or data analyst to save costs. We have requested 50% salary support for Dr.   's work on the study in year 03.

For the third year, Dr.   's participation will drop to 5%, since at that point, she will mainly be reviewing completed analyses and papers in preparation for publication. We anticipate that we will need the data coordinator for the first six months of year 03 to finish data entry and cleaning.

The administrative assistant will be needed to aid in administrative work to complete data collection, pay subjects and staff, and assist in the preparation of materials for publication and presentation. Salary support is requested for 50% for the administrative assistant also. Salary requests include performance advances and a 5% cost of living increase for all staff (except Dr.   , whose time is contributed).

Non-clinician interviewer costs for the third year will total $20,000 at $80 per interview for the remaining 250 follow-up interviews. Subject payment (at $25 per interview) will total $6,250. We have budgeted the same amount for travel and Dr.   's consultation (review of papers, at this point in the study) as in year 02.

General Issues of Feasibility, Quality Control, Cost Effectiveness

The Principal Investigator and the co-Principal Investigator have worked together for a number of years in a manner similar to that proposed in this application. Dr.   will take primary responsibility for the data collection and handling, consulting with Dr.   as needed. Dr.   has had extensive experience in recruiting subjects and retaining them in studies, many of which had complex designs requiring participation in more than one interview. Dr.   has demonstrated ability in this area as well.

Dr.   will work with Dr.   on adapting departmental procedures for this study, and organizationally integrating the work required for this project with the other ongoing studies in the department. Trained and experienced staff are already available in the department to work on the study if it is funded.

We have developed procedures for data tracking, checking, computerized editing, and rapid feedback to interviewers and protocol monitors. We are well aware of the importance of immediate editing and logging in of data once interviews have been completed. Computerized tracking of subjects will provide staff reminders of due dates for interviews, and information on which interviewers have previously interviewed subjects (information needed for the reliability and follow-up interviews). Past experience shows that our procedures ensure good quality control.

The establishment of the sample is a major expense in the proposed study, particularly reflected in the first-year budget. However, while we currently seek funds only for a short-term follow-up, we hope to re-assess subjects repeatedly over a period of several years, making the initial expense an investment in the gathering of future knowledge. Given the characteristics of the subjects and the nature of the data initially collected, we feel that this sample has the potential to yield a great deal of important information on the predictors of onset, chronicity and remission of alcohol dependence and related problems, and subgroups of the subjects may prove informative in later studies focused on aspects of alcohol dependence not covered in this initial application. In addition, we have designed the study to achieve a number of the different objectives outlined in the NIAAA RFA on nosology of alcohol use disorders. The fact that numerous components of the study can be carried out under the aegis of a single core administrative staff results in a more cost-effective procedure to achieve the research goals of the grant proposal than would be possible with several smaller studies that each required funds for their own administrative personnel. We note that the availability of free computer time, the lack of a need for a programmer/statistician, coverage of Dr.   's salary for a portion of the study, and the contribution of   funds for staff salaries and other expenses does serve to reduce the costs of the project somewhat.

Index